SELF-DISCIPLINE THROUGH IKIGAI AND KAIZEN

A MINDFUL APPROACH TO BUILD TINY HABITS AND MASTER YOUR FOCUS.

TWO BOOKS IN ONE.

BY

MARK MORIMOTO

ABOUT THE AUTHOR

Mark Morimoto is a self-help writer born and raised in California, always fascinated by his Japanese origins.

At the young age of 17 he went through a period of depression after the loss of his mother, suffering a lot because he believed he could not find a purpose in his life. But, thanks to his grandmother, he decided to take a path of rediscovery in his Japanese origins.

He moved to Japan, where he lived for 8 years. The discovery of Japanese philosophy applied in everyday life radically changed his perspective and his own life, which improved considerably.

Since then, he has embraced the mission of sharing the inestimable value of the small pearls of wisdom he learned in his experience.

He is the author of the books *Practical Guide to Ikigai. How to Find Purpose, Happiness, and Longevity Through Mini Habits, the Japanese Way,* and *Practical Guide to Kaizen. How to Reach Your Goals and Increase Your Productivity Through Mini Habits, the Japanese Way.* With these strategies, Mark has taught and motivated thousands to live a healthy and happier life.

Mark self-produces his own books. If you enjoy this book, please take a moment to provide your review. Just a little line or two will make a huge difference.

PRACTICAL GUIDE TO IKIGAI

HOW TO FIND PURPOSE, HAPPINESS, AND LONGEVITY THROUGH MINI HABITS, THE JAPANESE WAY

BY

MARK MORIMOTO

INTRODUCTION

Ikigai articulated [ikigai] is a Japanese concept that signifies "a reason for being." "Ikigai" is typically used to show the wellspring of significant worth in one's life or the things that make one's life advantageous. The word meant English generally signifies "thing that you live for" or "the explanation behind which you rise toward the beginning of the day." Every individual's ikigai is close to home to them and explicit to their lives, qualities, and convictions. It mirrors the internal identity of an individual and communicates that dependably while at the same time making a psychological state in which the individual feels calm. Exercises that permit one to contact ikigai are never constrained on an individual; they are frequently unconstrained and consistently attempted eagerly, giving the individual fulfillment and a feeling of importance to life.

The word ikigai, for the most part, is utilized to show the wellspring of significant worth in our life or things that make one's life beneficial. Furthermore, the word is used to allude to mental and profound conditions under which people feel that their lives are essential. It's not connected to one's monetary status. Regardless of whether an individual thinks that the present is dull; however, have an objective, they may feel ikigai. Practices that cause one to feel ikigai are not activities one is compelled to take—these are regular and unconstrained activities. Ikigai served its prime in Japan during the 1970s. It appears the concept has become one more common fare from the East, as a rule very withdrew from its unique, central importance in a considerable lot of the offered readings. In light of that, it may likewise appear to be anything but difficult to expel ikigai as a prevailing fashion, as another fare contorted and corrupted for the purpose.

There is a likely impact of having the sentiment of ikigai on the working of the prefrontal flap. It was factually demonstrated that the nearness of ikigai corresponds with a lower level of pressure and a general sentiment of being healthy. A few examinations indicated that individuals that don't feel ikigai are bound to encounter cardiovascular ailments; in any case, there was not discovered any relationship with the improvement of threatening tumors. The sentiment of ikigai adjusts the discharge of synapses, for example, dopamine, serotonin, and β-endorphin. A few examinations show that a feeling of purpose (objective) in life (ikigai) is contrarily connected with a requirement for endorsement from others and uneasiness. Concentrates additionally found that ikigai is related to the life span among Japanese individuals.

What number of us have thought, If I win this much, I'll be more joyful, or If I possessed that thing, I'd be more joyful? I'm willing to bet more than a couple. So it's reviving that lately, as a general public, we've begun to move away from the possibility that monetary achievement, riches, and assets are indications of accomplishment or the single things liable for our happiness. Instead, we're going to different nations and their unique concepts of happiness past riches. We've since a long time ago gone to yoga and reflection for finding an inside, and the abrupt furor for the Danish concept of hygge is another incredible case of this hunt. Various societies can offer an essential elective viewpoint on what happiness is or could be. They provide us bits of knowledge we may not, in any case, consider, and ikigai seems, by all accounts, to be the following concept to surprise us.

As per Japanese culture, everybody has ikigai. It shows the

worth that one finds in their life or the things that cause somebody to feel like their life is essential. It alludes to both mental and profound conditions that cause one to feel like their life has a reason. What truly sings for me about ikigai is that it's exchangeable. It's one of a kind to each person and recognizes that the possibility of "happiness" is entirely subtle. Ikigai, as a concept, can create as you do. If one way of purpose stops existing, you can adjust, change, and seek new interests with the aim. Ikigai prepares for this. There is a wide range of features to ikigai. However, there is one major part to it that genuinely stood apart for me. Even if your presence doesn't feel right, If you don't feel genuinely valuable in your present state yet, you have a reliable objective you're endeavoring towards; at that point, you will have discovered your ikigai.

As creatives, as and more than that — as ladies — we are so regularly the cause of all our problems. We contrast ourselves with others, and when we see people around us showing improvement over ourselves, we can feel like disappointments. We rapidly overlook what we are going after. We expel the excursion we're on. This is the place I think ikigai can serve genuine worth. If we follow the thoughts of ikigai, at that point, we're stepped back to ourselves, to our purpose, and the way that we're taking to arrive. Ikigai is as much about changes, challenges, and the missteps we may make, all things considered about "a definitive" accomplishment of a happy life.

The thought itself isn't notable or progressive, yet it merits observing. Eventually, ikigai isn't just about a long and upbeat life. It's tied in with recognizing the excursion you're on and making it your own, and comprehending what carries significance and purpose to your life at some random time.

It's about you.

CHAPTER ONE

THE CONCEPT OF IKIGAI

For some individuals, endeavoring to discover their purpose in life can take after a comparable winding mission, loaded up with numerous turns and wrong turns. Some aimlessly follow interests that aren't situated in actuality; at that point end up feeling disheartened when their fantasies don't emerge. Others surrender to vocations that bring them cash and status yet aren't satisfying. In the two cases, after some time, their feeling of purpose can start to blur.

What's more, as indicated by ongoing investigations, coming up short on a feeling of purpose can be impeding your health. One extensive examination found that individuals who have a sense of purpose in life are at lower danger of death and coronary illness. Why? Analysts found that individuals who feel purpose regularly have healthier lifestyles. They are increasingly spurred and durable, which shields them from stress and burnout. Analysts additionally found that while people from the U.S. characterized "purpose" as much the same as "value to other people," those from Japan were powered by a more profound, progressively broad translation of happiness. They allude to this as ikigai (articulate ee-kee-fellow).

What is ikigai?

Like the Danish word hygge, there's no straightforward, direct interpretation into English for the Japanese word ikigai. It generally implies "what you live for" or "the purpose behind which you find a good pace morning." more or less, it incorporates the possibility that happiness in life is about more than cash or an extravagant activity title.

In the post-pioneer, Western world, strict life has diminished considerably, energy has been supplanted with an across-the-board distrust of the legislature, and excelling has gotten exceedingly troublesome. Accordingly, an ever-increasing number of individuals are succumbing to apathy. This loathsome sentiment of harsh bafflement comes from the loss of importance in their lives.

An absence of purpose can expand the danger of psychological wellness issues, for example, nervousness and misery, bringing about more unfortunate rest, intensifying health, and in extraordinary cases, substance misuse and contemplations of suicide. Some have gone toward the East, most as of late, to the antiquated Japanese concept of ikigai, which implies, generally, "to live the acknowledgment one trusts in." Another understanding, "what makes life worth living." Take note that there's no definite English interpretation.

Iki signifies "life," though *gai* means "worth" or "worth." Gai originates from the word kai, signifying "shell." This alludes back to the Heian time frame (794 to 1185) when shells were viewed as necessary. We can decipher ikigai as discovering an incentive in one's life or finding one's purpose.

In the West, self-improvement masters and their developments have gone back and forth, and in the wake of each, however regularly lighter in the pocket, not many of their members discover genuine comfort. Maybe as opposed to happiness, which is commonly momentary and transitory, we should look for a purposeful life. Investigating the concept of ikigai and the inquiries that accompany it can assist one with finding a definite purpose and, through this, satisfaction and drive.

It's simplest to consider ikigai as a crossing point, the shared conviction between:

- What you love
- What you care about
- What the world needs
- What you can get paid for

Ikigai has a couple of essential characteristics that differentiate it from the "follow your enthusiasm" cliché as we consider it in Western culture:

- It's difficult. Your ikigai should prompt dominance and development.
- It's your decision. You feel a specific level of self-governance and opportunity-seeking after your ikigai.
- It includes the responsibility of time and conviction, maybe to a specific reason, aptitude, exchange, or gathering of individuals.

It helps your prosperity. Ikigai is related to positive connections and excellent health. It gives you more vitality than it removes.

In some sense, an ikigai can fill in as a compass to explore both vocation and life decisions, which it appears individuals desire until further notice like never before. 20% of twenty to thirty-year-olds and 21% of Gen-X's state that accomplishing work they are enthusiastic about is a significant long haul objective. Before you think this sounds too pure fantasy, consider what one scientist noted: ikigai is regularly not something terrific or unprecedented. What better way, at that point, to find an economic enthusiasm than by finding your ikigai?

Ikigai is a term that epitomizes the possibility of happiness in living. For Japanese specialists in substantial urban communities, an ordinary workday starts with a state called sushi-time, a time which compares suburbanites crushed into a jam-packed train vehicle to firmly pressed grains of rice in sushi. The pressure doesn't stop there. The nation's infamous work culture guarantees the vast majority put in extended periods at the workplace, represented by severe progressive standards. The exhaust isn't phenomenal, and the keep going trains home on weekdays around midnight are loaded up with individuals in suits. How would they oversee? The mystery may have to do with what the Japanese call ikigai. There is no immediate English interpretation, yet it's a term that typifies the possibility of happiness in living. Ikigai is the motivation behind why you find a workable pace morning.

In case you're resigned, you might not need to stress over what you can be paid for, so you can erase that one and spotlight on the staying three. The thought isn't just to discover your purpose, yet the correct harmony between all viewpoints encompassing it. Another idea, one's ikigai doesn't influence the individual alone. For the Japanese, the concept has a social component. It's tied in with getting settled with your job in your family, employment, and society. It's traditionally part of sexual orientation lines. While men usually partner their ikigai with their work and vocation, ladies (in any event traditionally) partner it with parenthood and their job in the family. Also, Even though ikigai has as of late become the most recent New Age popular expression in the West, this doesn't make it any less compelling for the individuals who wind up at a junction, with no sign to control them.

The Definition of Ikigai

There's no immediate interpretation of ikigai into English, yet the most precise definitions I've found are the accompanying:

- The term ikigai is made out of *iki* and *kai*. At present, kai is commonly written in hiragana (Japanese phonetic syllabary)… Iki alludes to 'life'; kai is an additional meaning generally 'the acknowledgment of what one expects and trusts in.
- Japanese word references characterize ikigai in such terms as *ikiru hariai, yorokobi,* meat (something to live for, the joy and objective of living)

This is genuinely near how Wikipedia depicts it too:

- The term ikigai mixes two Japanese words: *iki* meaning life, alive, and *kai* meaning '(an) impact; (a) result; (an) organic product; (a) value; (an) utilization; (a) benefit; profit' (successively voiced as *gai)* to show up at 'a purpose behind living; a significance for life; what makes life worth living.

One can likewise observe ikigai interpreted as:

- "reason for being"
- "The explanation behind which you get up in the first part of the day."
- "The direct interpretation is the 'happiness of being occupied.

In the wake of rehashing the bolded zones above, consider the possibility that we were to see ikigai like this.

Moment of clarity: Your "explanation behind being" gives you "motivation to live."

To the extent portrayals go, here are a couple I reverberate with:

- The procedure of permitting the self's prospects to bloom." (Note: This is significantly progressively powerful If you envision the ikigai diagram as a flower blossoming)
- "This word (ikigai) is genuinely similar to a fortune map. Furthermore, this fortune guide can assist you in finding your approach to finding brilliant things about yourself that you can impart to the world, and the world will say 'thank you for it."

To those in the West who are increasingly acquainted with the concept of ikigai, it's regularly connected with a Venn diagram with four covering characteristics: what you love, what you are acceptable at. For Japanese notwithstanding, the thought is marginally extraordinary. In an overview of 2,000 Japanese people directed, only 31% of beneficiaries considered work as their ikigai. Somebody's incentive in life can be work – yet is not restricted to that.

A More Intensive Look

In an examination paper on ikigai, co-creator Akihiro Hasegawa, a clinical analyst and partner teacher at Toyo Eiwa University, set the word ikigai as a feature of the ordinary Japanese language. It is made out of two words: *iki*, which implies life, and *gai*, which depicts worth or worth.

As indicated by Hasegawa, the beginning of the phrase ikigai returns to the Heian time frame (794 to 1185). "Gai originates from the word kai ("shell" in Japanese), which were considered exceptionally important, and from that point, ikigai is inferred as a word that implies an incentive in living."

There are different words that utilization *kai*: *yarigai* or *hatarakigai*, which means the benefit of doing and the benefit of working. Ikigai can be thought of as a broad concept that joins such qualities in life. There are numerous books in Japan committed to ikigai. However, one is explicitly viewed as complete: Ikigai-ni-tsuite (About Ikigai), distributed in 1966.

Ikigai is like "happiness"; however, an unpretentious difference in its subtlety has. Ikigai is the thing that permits you to anticipate the future regardless of whether you're hopeless at this moment. Japanese individuals accept that the total of small joys in regular day-to-day existence brings about an additionally satisfying life all in all. It is brought up that in English, the word life implies both lifetime and regular daily existence. In this way, ikigai interpreted as life's purpose sounds exceptionally fantastic. "Be that as it may, in Japan we have *jinsei*, which implies lifetime, and *seikatsu*, which implies regular day-to-day existence," he says. The concept of ikigai adjusts more to *seikatsu*, and, through his exploration, Hasegawa found that Japanese individuals accept that the aggregate of small joys in regular daily existence brings about an additionally satisfying life all in all.

It was firmly identified with the expression "*chanto sure*," or doing things appropriately. The concept of ikigai is entirely defined with the Japanese island of Okinawa, whose occupants enjoy a fantastic life span. Many centenarians can be found there, and some acknowledge finding their ikigai for long, healthy life. One restriction is, If one considers there to be as their ikigai, they may disregard their family, companions, and pastimes, which are similarly as significant and satisfying. Also, the Japanese themselves are thinking that it's hard to accomplish ikigai. Pretty much 31% of Japanese respondents said they'd discovered theirs in a study directed. What's more, If you achieve yours, is that the end? The individuals who have an away from of ikigai can accomplish higher parts of comprehension past it, for example, "*ittaikan*" or a feeling of unity with one's social job, and "*jiko jitsugen*" or self-acknowledgment.

A Concept for Life Span?

Japan has probably the longest-living residents on the planet – 87 years for ladies and 81 for men, as indicated by the nation's Ministry of Health, Labor, and Welfare. Could this concept of ikigai add to the life span? Exercises on Living Longer from the People Who've Lived the Longest, and has ventured to every part of the globe investigating seemingly perpetual networks far and wide, which he calls "blue zones." One such zone is Okinawa, a remote island with an astoundingly high number of centenarians. While one of a kind eating regimen likely has a great deal to do with inhabitants' life span, says ikigai additionally has an impact. More established individuals are praised; they feel committed to give their astuteness to younger ages.

The concept of ikigai isn't restrictive to Okinawans: there probably won't be a word for it yet in each of the four blue zones, for example, Sardinia and the Nicoya Peninsula, a similar concept exists among individuals living long lives. We recommend making three records: your qualities, things you like to do, and things you are acceptable at. The cross-segment of the three documents is your ikigai. Be that as it may, knowing your ikigai alone isn't sufficient. You need an outlet. Ikigai is a purpose in real life. For a 92-year-elderly person, her ikigai may be to move and sing with her friends in the KBG84 move troupe. For other people, it may be work itself.

In a culture where the estimation of the group supersedes the individual, Japanese specialists are driven by being helpful to other people, being expressed gratitude toward, and being regarded by their partners. If you need to begin an organization, however, you are frightened to jump into the obscure, take a quick trip, and see somebody who is, as of now, planning something comparative for what you have at the top of the priority list. Observing your arrangements in real life will give you the certainty that you can do it as well.

Think Smaller

Saying this doesn't imply that working harder and longer are fundamental principles of the ikigai theory – about a fourth of Japanese representatives work over 80 hours of extra time a month, and with lamentable results – the wonder of karoshi (passing from exhaust) asserts more than 2,000 lives every year. Or maybe, ikigai is tied in with feeling your work has any kind of effect on individuals' lives. How individuals discover importance in their work is a subject of a lot essential to the executive's specialists. One research clarified that what rouses representatives is "accomplishing work that influences the prosperity of others" and to "see or meet the individuals influenced by their work."

In a trial, time was gone through with a beneficiary of the grant they were attempting to fund-raise for acquired 171%

more cash when contrasted and the individuals who were just working the telephone. The necessary demonstration of meeting an understudy recipient gave importance to the pledge drives and helped their presentation. This applies to life as a rule. Rather than attempting to handle world yearning, you can begin small by helping somebody around you, similar to a neighborhood chipping in a gathering.

Differentiate your Ikigai

Retirement can bring an immense feeling of misfortune and void for the individuals who discover their ikigai in work. This can be particularly valid for competitors, who have generally shorter vocations. Champion hurdler Dai Tamesue, who resigned in 2012, said that the essential inquiry he posed after he left was: "what was it that I needed to accomplish by playing sports?"

"For me, what I needed to accomplish through contending in Olympic-style events was to change individuals' recognitions." In the wake of resigning, he began an organization that supports sports-related business. Every one of these shows the moldable idea of ikigai and how it very well may be applied. At the point when retirement comes, it is useful to have an away from of why you do what you do past gathering a payslip. By being aware of this concept, it may very well assist you with living an all the more satisfying life.

Ikigai Myths: Three Big Misperceptions of Ikigai in the West

1. Ikigai isn't identified with work or cash

Ikigai isn't really about your work (you weren't destined to work): In an overview of 2,000 Japanese people directed by Central Research Services in 2010, only 31% of beneficiaries considered work as their ikigai. Somebody's incentive in life can be work – yet is not constrained to that. There is proof in the way that numerous Japanese individuals keep seeking after their ikigai until the finish of their lives: Many Japanese individuals never honestly resign. In essence, they continue doing what they love for whatever length of time that their health permits.

Ikigai can be family, a fantasy, or basically, the profound inclination that life merits living. Ikigai might be imagined either as the 'object' that causes one's life to appear to merit living (ikigai taishō) — one's work or family or dream—or as the inclination that experience merits living (ikigai kan). The word 'ikigai' is typically used to demonstrate the wellspring of significant worth in one's life or the things that make one's life beneficial (for instance, one may state: 'This kid is my ikigai'). Also, the word is utilized to allude to mental and profound conditions under which people feel that their lives are significant.

This is a significant difference contrasted with different models for life purposes. Your purpose doesn't need to be attached to your vocation. I have numerous companions who revealed to me they realized they were intended to have youngsters before they even comprehended what it was to imagine. I've generally accepted that tolerating the call to be a mother is the decision to turn into a definitive profound educator since moms live in administration and penance to their youngsters.

Normally, If your ikigai doesn't need to be business-related, at that point, cash can (and should) be expelled from the diagram. Alongside the observation that ikigai identifies with work, the hover for "that which you can be paid for" gets a ton of analysis for being a confusion by Westerners. Finding the appropriate responses and harmony between these four territories could be a course to ikigai for Westerners searching for a fast understanding of this way of thinking. Yet, in Japan, ikigai is a more slow procedure and regularly has nothing to accomplish with work or play.

Ikigai gives people a feeling of a life worth living. It isn't identified with financial status. Practices that cause one to feel ikigai are not activities that people are compelled to take. However, they are unconstrained exercises that individuals attempt eagerly. Ikigai is close to home; it mirrors the internal identity of an individual and communicates that steadfastly. It sets up an extraordinary mental world in which the individual can feel quiet. Some accept this could be reframed as "what you can be compensated for."

2. Ikigai doesn't need to be seen as a mind-boggling, win significant or bust life purpose

There's no lack of individuals out there who need to persuade you that you have one life purpose and one life purpose as it were. This can be extraordinarily overpowering for individuals as they attempt to locate their unrivaled object.

What I've discovered is that: Ikigai isn't something fantastic or phenomenal. It's something matter-of-truth. — Gordon Mathews, educator of humanities. You don't require an enormous desire to be cheerful; you simply need a lot of companions to drink green tea and talk with. Dispose of the wreckage and at the center is your ikigai. It's about the procedure versus the last point: I have learned in my exploration with more seasoned Japanese, what makes ikigai powerful is it's inseparable connect to a feeling of dominance

– the thought known as *'chanto sure'* that things ought to be done appropriately. Ikigai accentuates procedure and drenching as opposed to the last point.

3. One can possess more than one ikigai in your life

One thing to remember is that you can alter your life purpose at any age. Usually, your use will advance after some time: They have a significant purpose in life or a few. They have an ikigai. However, they don't pay attention to it as well. They are loose and enjoy all that they do.

In the wake of talking loads of centenarians and supercentenarians in Ogimi, Okinawa to attempt to comprehend their life theory and life span insider facts, many built up their ten guidelines of ikigai:

1. Stay dynamic; don't resign.
2. Take it moderately.
3. Don't fill your stomach.
4. Surround yourself with old buddies.
5. Get fit as a fiddle for your next birthday.
6. Smile.
7. Reconnect with nature.
8. Give much obliged.
9. Live at the time.
10. Follow your ikigai.

CHAPTER TWO

THE IKIGAI DIAGRAM FOR LIFE PURPOSE

All things considered, in the remainder of the world, many inquired about these locales and named them the 'Blue Zones.' Japan and the island Okinawa specifically are such a district. A significant factor in the health and essentialness of Okinawa inhabitants is to have 'an objective' in their lives: 'ikigai.' So notwithstanding dietary patterns and living conditions, this Japanese concept assumes a significant job in maturing healthily since your 'ikigai' makes it conceivable to continue looking towards the future, in any event, when you are experiencing a troublesome time.

Ikigai has double importance. If you somehow happened to summarize the different definitions and can them, we could arrange them like this (reworded):

1. The inclination/profound implying that life merits living (being): Universal human experience, the happiness, and benefit of being alive, people as otherworldly creatures, the joy of living, feeling that life is essential/worth living

2. The wellspring of significant worth in one's life that merits living for (doing): Things that make one's life advantageous, something to live for, developing one's internal potential, permitting the self's prospects to bloom, one's work or family or dream, the acknowledgment of what one expects and trusts in

I accept the most potent ikigai adjusts both of these:

Ikigai Dual Meaning = Life merits living (being) and worth

living for (doing).

This is the complete fundamental piece that practically the entirety of the excellent ways to deal with life purpose forget about: BEING.

"The consistent idea among them: They have found that right now, is no genuine managing without first being."

Oprah helped put otherworldly instructor Eckhart Tolle on the standard guide. Tolle clarifies why being is essential and must precede doing. It turns out the ikigai double importance is actually what Eckhart Tolle educates:

- The most significant thing to acknowledge is this: Your life has an internal purpose and an external purpose. Inward mission concerns Being and is essential. Foreign object concerns doing and is optional.
- Doing is rarely enough If you disregard Being. The sense of self remains unaware of yet trusting you will, in the long run, be spared by doing. If you are in the hold of the knowledge of self, you accept that by accomplishing increasingly more, you will find in the long-run aggregate enough 'doings' to cause yourself to feel total sooner or later. You won't. You will just lose yourself in doing it. The whole human progress is losing itself in doing that isn't established in being and accordingly gets purposeless.
- Your internal purpose is to stir. It is as basic as that. You share that purpose individually on the planet – because it is the purpose of humanity.

Your inward goal is an essential piece of the meaning of the entire universe and its rising knowledge.

- Awakened doing is the arrangement of your external purpose¬ (what you do) with your internal purpose (arousing and remaining wakeful).

Ikigai Diagram

'Ikigai' is a Japanese concept that signifies 'your motivation to get up toward the beginning of the day.' In French, it is called 'raison d'être.' Ikigai is a blend of the words '*iki*', which implies life or living, and the word '*kai*' (articulated as gai), which speaks to esteem, impact, result, or convenience.

What is 'ikigai' precisely? It is that place where your energy, strategy, and profession converge. This is best represented by the covering circles of a Venn diagram.

The four circles speak to:

1. What you love
2. What you are acceptable at
3. What the world needs
4. What you are/could be paid for

Where the four circles meet is the place you discover your 'ikigai.'

Step by step Instructions to Apply your Ikigai

You can just apply your 'ikigai' when you realize what it is going after for some individuals that requires a full pursuit of the self-first. However, If you need to make a beginning at comprehension of your 'ikigai,' you could begin by making your own Venn diagram. Fill the circles with words, thoughts, pictures, or sentences that fall under the 'You like it,' 'You are acceptable at it,' 'The world needs it,' and 'you are paid for it.'

Attempt to respond to addresses like What makes you tick?; What contacts you?; What are you acceptable at?; Which exceptional gifts do you have, and which would you be able to additionally create?; What would you be able to do that is useful to other people?; What change might you want to achieve on the planet? Quest for the (standard) cover of the different circles. Take a gander at the total picture and attempt to discover associations. If you do it, take as much time as is needed. Give thoughts and driving forces an opportunity and keep a receptive outlook. That way, your 'ikigai' will, in the long run, become apparent.

Points of Interest in Having an Ikigai

The upsides of having an 'ikigai' appear to be precise. It gives you the motivation to find a workable pace morning. You are enjoying in your work, adoring what you do, and offering importance to your reality. Joined with healthy eating and a decent living condition, your 'ikigai' is a significant element for healthy maturing.

Ikigai Model

In a quickly evolving world, an ever-increasing number of individuals are searching for an approach to consolidate their enthusiasm and abilities to add to society. That is fundamentally what 'ikigai' is. An engaging case of individuals who practice their 'ikigai' consistently is David de Kock and Arjan Vergeer from 365 days fruitful. They mean to make the Netherlands the most joyful nation on the planet, and they need to accomplish that by helping other people get the best out of themselves. As it's been said on their site: 'One thing we learned as of late: If you truly need something and you pick a technique to arrive, the sky is the limit. In your brain, however particularly as a general rule.'

Ikigai is a Japanese concept that is tied in with having (of finding) an objective in life, a purpose behind getting up in the first part of the day. Your 'ikigai' is where various perspectives meet up, to be specific what you love, what you are acceptable at, what the world needs, and what you can be paid for. It is the place for your energy, strategy, and calling the meeting. The reason for finding your 'ikigai' is typically a broad quest for yourself.

Finding Your Life's Meaning with The Discover of Ikigai Diagram

What's the importance of life? No, extremely: what's the significance of your life? It's a well-established inquiry, yet you could contend that it's the establishment of genuine life-long happiness, satisfaction, and even self-realization. Arriving, be that as it may, may take a lifetime of work!

To speed that along with a piece, I offer "ikigai," a Japanese concept I ran over. Actually deciphered, ikigai signifies "purpose behind being": "Ikiru" means "to live," and "kai" signifies "the acknowledgment of what one trusts in." Paraphrased, it's the explanation you find a workable pace! When I read a little increasingly about ikigai, I perceive how the concept can incorporate – without a doubt amplify – an individual's expert, individual, otherworldly, and passionate life. As leaders, as experts, as individuals: we're all making progress toward balance – we're all taking a stab at purpose, happiness, and satisfaction. So as we wind down summer and apparatus up for what I'm sure will be a bustling fall for a large portion of us, I offer these experiences to assist you with finding your ikigai – your actual importance in life.

Ikigai is a concept – a system, a model – that has four crucial inquiries that cover into a Venn diagram:

1.   What do you love?
2.   At what are you accept?
3.   What does the world need from you? Furthermore,
4.   For what would you be able to get paid?

We Should Investigate Each.

What do you love? The primary inquiry is maybe the most effortless to reply. Think about your leisure activities; consider what unwinds or restores you, of what gives you vitality. Perhaps it's planting, or wellness and working out, or cooking, or photography, voyaging, perusing sports, specialties, creatures, or any number of things. It could be identified with your work, your family, your volunteer exercises, as well as your advantages. I'm sure the majority of us know the answer(s) to this inquiry directly, all things being equal; however, If you need assistance, there are a couple of excellent articles and assets out there to invigorate your reasoning.

At what are you accept? The subsequent inquiry identifies with your aptitudes and skills – they can surely be proficient (identified with what you accomplish busy working). However, they could likewise be close to home (possibly you're acceptable at finishing, or drawing, or singing, or recounting stories, or any number of things). There are additionally some fantastic assets – like Strengths Finder –

that can assist you with distinguishing stuff at which you exceed expectations. Furthermore, this is something you can create after some time – with extra proper instruction, at work or study hall preparing, affirmations, stretch assignments, etc. If what you love meets with your qualities (questions 1 and 2), at that point, ikigai says that you have discovered your passion(s). For instance, If you love planting and you're acceptable at cultivating, your energy is growing!

What does the world need from you? Question three is tied in with finding what the world needs. If the world needs plant specialists and you love to plant, you discovered your lives strategically. Despite what might be expected, if there are an excessive number of plant specialists as of now – or if the world simply needn't bother with cultivators – you may need to investigate other world requires that you love doing to find that strategy. There are various assets to help all of us answer this inquiry. I would recommend starting with a look into occupations that are sought after or that are enjoying anticipated high development. Rising fields or rising innovation. And new items and arrangements that address human needs (none of us realized that we required another transportation strategy until Uber was conceived, and now there are a vast number of Uber drivers needed for the world, and a considerable lot of them love to drive!).

For what would you be able to get paid? What's more, the last inquiry identifies with what the world is happy to pay you for doing – a market, maybe. If individuals need a plant specialist and they are eager to pay you to plant for them, you found a job. If they're willing to pay you for planting and you're great at it (question 2), you discovered your calling. Entirely clear up until this point, I'm sure. Be that as it may, there are five new convergences in the ikigai model that are truly uncovering:

- If what you love is what you're acceptable at and the world is happy to pay you for it, yet it's honestly not what the world needs, you have fulfillment, yet a sentiment of pointlessness. It's elusive models for this, yet perhaps it's a performer or a jokester. You love doing it, might be acceptable at it, and individuals are eager to pay for it. However, it honestly doesn't fill quite a bit of a need.

- If what you love doing is the thing that the world needs and is happy to pay for, yet you're not excellent at it, you'll feel fervor and smugness, however, a feeling of vulnerability. Alright – this is me playing golf! I love doing it (more often than not). The world needs it (I surmise) and is eager to pay for it (passes to competitions, TV commercials, and so on.) – however, I'm simply not sufficient to cause a to go at it expertly. I'd sure be eager to attempt to be an expert golf player, yet I'd have an immense feeling of vulnerability, realizing that my absence of aptitudes would, in the end, this mission.

- If what you love doing is something you're acceptable at and something the world needs yet isn't happy to pay for, at that point, you'll have pleasure and totality, however, no riches. This crossing point may be a decent possibility for charitable effort – satisfying inside and out; however, it doesn't get you a check.

- If what you're acceptable at is something the world needs and is happy to pay for, yet you genuinely don't cherish doing it, you'll be agreeable, however, have a sentiment of vacancy. I'm speculating numerous callings fit this portrayal – you accomplish great work, you get your check. Yet, you're genuinely not too satisfied. Check-in; get paid; return home, and do whatever it is you truly enjoy.

Those four convergences in the model leave you halfway unfulfilled and presumably speak to reality for some (most?) of us in the Western world.

In any case, the fifth convergence – where everything covers in the model – speaks to a perfect state. If what you love doing is something you're acceptable at doing and something the world needs and what you can be paid for, you've found ikigai – your actual life's purpose and meaning, and harmony between what you can (and need to) do that is of incentive to the world. To start to find your ikigai, I would recommend you ponder those four essential inquiries – may be utilizing a portion of the devices and assets I referenced above and maybe emphasizing them over some time. My sense is there isn't one ideal response for every one of the four inquiries, yet rather a moving continuum of choices that, when joined, produce a corresponding equalization – something that moves toward the center of the Venn diagram.

In any case, simply knowing your ikigai isn't sufficient: you should place your life's purpose vigorously. If you find you're out of parity (at the end of the day, you're encountering one of those four situations above in slugs, where a few of the inquiries cover yet the awkwardness prompts sentiments of futility, vacancy, absence of riches, or vulnerability), at that point, you ought to investigate changes – either in your vocation, in your instruction and expert advancement, or both. What you love to do and what the world needs may move after some time; what you're acceptable at and what you can be paid for (your job/calling) are the factors over which you have the most control. So your activity ought to identify with bettering your aptitudes and additionally changing your vocation, so your enthusiasm, crucial, and job are in arrangement.

Genuine North is your situating point – your fixed point in a turning world – that encourages you to remain on target as a pioneer. It is gotten from your most profoundly held convictions, your qualities, and the standards you lead by. It is your inside compass, interesting to you, that speaks to who you are at your most profound level. Many battles that finding your True North – like finding your ikigai – will make you legitimate, the authentic you. It's the sweet detect that incorporates your own life, proficient life, family life, and network and companions. It's the convergence of your qualities, your purpose, and your locale. It sounds sort of like ikigai.

As leaders, as experts, as individuals, you owe it to your association, your group, your family, and yourself to discover your life's actual significance and purpose. We, as a whole, ought to be on a steady journey to locate our ikigai!

Why and How the Ikigai Diagram Needs to be Redesigned (Five Key Points)

Given that the first diagram was only a concept for life purpose and not straightforwardly identified with ikigai, we should begin without any preparation. We'll leave that venture for one more day and somewhat adjust and advance what the world knows as the "ikigai diagram.

Here are five key focuses illustrating why and how I think the ikigai diagram should be refreshed:

1. WHY: We require the ikigai model to join both being and doing.

This is shrouded in the introduction of this post.

HOW: It is accepted that this should be outwardly reflected in the focal point of the diagram. Being and doing must be adjusted together.

2. WHY: We have to re-calibrate the model to more precisely portray the truth of Japanese ikigai versus the Westernized interpretation.

What does the Blue Zones region say about ikigai?

- Individuals who comprehend what brings them joy and happiness will, in general, have what we like to call the Right Outlook. They are overwhelmed in exercises and networks that permit them to drench themselves in a fulfilling and satisfying condition.
- Do an interior stock—consider your beliefs, standards, benchmarks, and ethics. At that point, think about your physical, enthusiasm, and mental gifts, qualities, and capacities.

HOW: We have to fuse Right Outlook into the model. I accept gifts/standards/goals that fall into the current circles.

3. WHY: We need the ikigai diagram to expel cash as a prerequisite.

This is shrouded in more detail in the past ikigai post If you need a boost. Numerous individuals in Okinawa never "resign." They play out their ikigai (or have different purposes) for whatever length of time that they live. A few people have an ikigai identified with their family, which additionally underpins why cash ought to be evacuated.

<u>HOW</u>: Remove the hover for "what you can be paid for" and show cash as a discretionary side-effect/result of living your ikigai (pertinent for a few; for nobody else).

<u>4. WHY</u>: The diagram needs to show that ikigai is about the procedure versus the last point.

Ikigai underlines procedure, drenching, and a feeling of authority as opposed to an ultimate objective:

- You don't ascend to the degree of your goals. You tumble to the degree of your frameworks.
- It is your promise to the procedure that will decide your advancement.
- The procedure proceeds until the end of time:
- I think life is a procedure. You wake up. At that point, you wake up some more. Oneself bites the dust. Another is conceived. It's an advancement of cognizance.

<u>HOW</u>: We need a visual component that shows that there is a progressing procedure engaged with ikigai.

<u>5. WHY</u>: We need the ikigai diagram to represent the need request/weighting.

This works two different ways:

- Clockwise around the diagram: Each progression is a channel for the earlier circle
- Example 1: I love music, yet I'm not encoded for it. This doesn't work.

- Example 2: If you love something and are encoded for it, this could go to egocentricity or covetousness if not separated through what the world needs. In principle, If you are doing twisted with being, this shouldn't prompt a position of narrow-mindedness/insatiability in any case. However, circle 3 is another checkpoint here and permits you to outline what you do in the setting of the world/humankind.
- Counterclockwise around the diagram:
- Example 1: Being hereditarily encoded for something isn't sufficient If you don't adore it enough to do anything with it.
- Example 2: You can disregard what the world needs If you can't make sense of what you need.

<u>HOW</u>: Show that there is a need for request/weighting by changing the size of the circles in like manner and show that the procedure is to tail them clockwise.

What's The Difference Between the Purpose Diagram and Ikigai?

If you aren't a hermit, you've most likely observed various variants of the purpose diagram skimming around the web. The two most popular forms either have purpose or ikigai on the inside. In case you're pondering about the starting point of the diagram. To put it plainly, the purpose diagram started things out, and afterward, a splendid individual named Marc Winn joined my purpose diagram with the Japanese concept of ikigai. The purpose diagram had just turned into a web trend; however, once ikigai was set in the inside, it spread quickly: ikigai instructive offers, ikigai shirts, ikigai workshops, ikigai diaries, and books showed up all over the place. The most notable among them was about talking with Japanese centenarians and situating ikigai as the mystery prompting their life span.

For What Reason did Ikigai Take off far Beyond Purpose?

This is a splendid case of the power of showcasing. The ubiquity of thoughts depends a great deal more on the story you can tell around it. What's more, recounting the narrative of an antiquated Japanese concept that we can gain from in the 21st century is a lot hotter than the exceptionally rational, thus generally philosophized term "purpose." We, as a whole, love modern concepts, and giving a different take to an old one feels both tradition-regarding, built up, to be trusted, and newly restless simultaneously.

Try not to misunderstand me! I love the Aikikai thought, and I praise the spreading of the concept. Anything that gets individuals to change from a hopeless work trench to addressing why they are living their life how they are gets a high five from me. Be that as it may, I'm not an enthusiast of calling the diagram ikigai, and here is the reason: Working with the four-circle diagram and calling it ikigai captures Japanese culture. The purpose diagram (those named four covering circles) has nothing to do with the Japanese expression ikigai. If you demonstrated the description to a shrewd Japanese centenarian, they would likely be extremely confounded.

According to clinical therapist Akihiro Hasegawa and his 2001 research paper, the term ikigai goes back to the Heian time frame (794 to 1185) and is made out of two words: *iki*, meaning life and gain portraying worth or worth. (For the historical underpinnings nerds, *gai* originates from *kai*, which means shell, which was entirely crucial at that point.) Today, ikigai is a piece of ordinary language. Be that as it may, learn to expect the unexpected. The Japanese concept of Ikigai isn't about your terrific life's purpose. It's about the little things. If you take a gander at the traditional writing on ikigai, you'll locate a 1966 piece called *Ikigai-ni-tsuite* ("About Ikigai") by specialist Mieko Kamika. He clarifies the subtleties of ikigai. There are two sorts of "life" in the Japanese language: *jinsei* and *seikatsu*. As per him, *jinsei* alludes to lifetime, and seikatsu alludes to regular day-to-day existence. Ikigai lines up with *seikatsu*, for example, regular daily existence and is about the aggregate of small joys in ordinary daily existence that lead to an all the more satisfying life in general.

This is what ikigai isn't about: work, boosting what you're getting paid while amplifying your joy, effect, and aptitudes, which happens to be what the purpose diagram is about.

Presently before the business mentors who have fabricated their site around ikigai have a tantrum: YES! Indeed, you CAN discover the joy in your life and live as per cigar AND have a vocation that you love, that you're acceptable at, in which you increase the value of the world and are liberally paid for. Be that as it may, ikigai, as indicated by Japanese culture, isn't something you have to bring in cash from, doesn't need to be something the world needs, isn't something you must be especially profoundly gifted at, and you don't need to adore doing it.

The purpose diagram is a Western way of thinking, and keeping in mind that I can't clarify any other individual methods when they use it, I can let you know with which expectation I apply it. I made my adaptation of the purpose diagram as an analytic preview device for individuals to figure out where they believe themselves to be inside their professions. Am I having contact with what I do? Am I enjoying how I invest my energy? Do I find good pace things I know, and do I find excellent pace abilities I need to advance? Am I content with the amount I'm getting paid? The procedure that I instruct in enormous corporate associations and train the mentor courses assists associations with coordinating individuals' personal feelings of professional purpose with their group's mission and the bigger authoritative purpose.

The purpose diagram and the business related to it are especially about purpose in real life. The picture helps leaders, singular vocation entertainers, and business people to comprehend how everything fits in together and what they need to be more on purpose.

Calling the Diagram Ikigai Makes it Challenging to Offer to Leaders and Decision-Makers

Despite being a rather interesting story, the anecdote of ikigai and the beliefs of Japanese culture regarding the representation and estimation of life put the discussion around purpose in a crate marked B.A.C. This translates to a "wonderful ancient concept that you can dig into when secretly considering how to invest more energy with your friends and family, do the little things that bring you joy, and carry on with a life of zero second thoughts." It doesn't help with persuading a CEO to reexamine professional structures, chip away at giving groups what they need to cooperate all the most adequately and assist individuals with gaining a feeling of arrangement between their occupation and what the association is doing deliberately.

That is actually what the world needs: more associations that exist for some reasons past benefit and leaders who apply the cover of the components of the diagram - sway, which means joy and gainfulness - at all degrees of their association. The corporate purpose might be en route to turning into a popular expression; however, we, despite everything, need approaches to operationalize the goal; what's more, to do that, we need a corporate-good language for it. The expression "ikigai" basically doesn't work well for that specific purpose (joke expected).

Calling the purpose diagram ikigai makes it sound theoretical as opposed to relevant. A few people know about the previous factors and still kindness the term ikigai. They believe they can consciously explain the absence of connection between the diagram and Japanese culture, and maybe they don't require business-perfect language in their specific field of work. Be that as it may, an issue endures: our human propensity to search for arrangements out there instead of within us. At the point when we utilize a term that is theoretical to most non-Japanese individuals, it upholds the thought that we should look for answers and comprehend a tricky unique answer that is in the distance. What's more, that, when we discover it, everything will bode well and become all-good. Spoiler alert: it won't.

This equivalent human component is the thing that causes leaders to present profitability framework after efficiency framework (KANBAN, OGSTs, OKRs and so forth.), procure the concurring mentors and pay for the important programming, as opposed to discussing the conflicts of various kinds of requirements of various people and their correspondence inclinations. Team profitability, much like group purpose, is an inside activity that expects us to look at our world straight in the eye and discussion about what isn't working. To me, the purpose isn't a goal; however, a work in progress, a ceaseless condition of lasting beta.

Thus, regardless of the bigger ubiquity of the term ikigai, I have decided to continue working with the first wording purpose because:

1. The term purpose is vigorous and direct. When something stops having a purpose in our life, we, for the most part, let it go or figure out how to change it. That is a straightforward and powerful affiliation.
2. The concept of purpose can undoubtedly be moved to corporate reality. "What is the purpose of this group and association?" causes us to center around noteworthy inquiries that issue for associations that need to turn out to be more purpose-driven.
3. "Purpose" is a significant word that can trigger obstruction. I'm a fanatic of making statements as they are, and utilizing "purpose" is satisfactory because it mirrors the truth (at whatever point you work with transform, you will undoubtedly face individual and foundational opposition) and because the obstruction is the rich issue that you can work with, as an individual and with your groups and association.

If you love the way of thinking of ikigai and Japanese culture, set out to find out about its actual birthplace and address neighborhood specialists. In case you're searching for an instrument to bring more purpose into your/an association's work reality, work with the purpose diagram.

CHAPTER THREE

THE MOST IMPORTANT PILLARS OF IKIGAI AND THEIR BENEFITS

The concept of Ikigai begins in Japan and has gotten mainstream around the globe in the previous barely any years. Notwithstanding helping you live a longer and physically, and intellectually healthier life, finding your Ikigai will likewise feel you satisfied and centered in your work. It causes you to feel energetic about your objectives and assist you with living and work with respectability. Seeking after your purpose can likewise give you an expanded sentiment of self-esteem since you see that you increase the value of the world. Notwithstanding, the premise of Ikigai is that it doesn't simply advance your own life, however that of others also.

In Japan, the key to living a longer, more joyful, and progressively satisfying life can be summarized in a single word: Ikigai. This belief system dates to the Heian time frame (A.D. 794 to 1185), yet just in the previous decade has it gained consideration from millions around the globe. The cigar lifestyle is particularly conspicuous in Okinawa, in a gathering of islands south of territory Japan. (It has additionally been nicknamed the "Place where there are Immortals" since it has among the longest lifespans and most noteworthy paces of centenarians on the planet.)

'The purpose behind which you get up in the first part of the day.'

The lifestyle qualities of five places on the planet where individuals live the longest.: of all the blue zones,

Okinawans have the most noteworthy life anticipation.

In America, grown-up life is isolated into two classifications: Our work life and our retirement life," he says. "In Okinawa, there isn't even a word for retirement. Rather there's basically 'ikigai,' which signifies 'the explanation behind which you get up toward the beginning of the day. The ikigai of a few Okinawans: For a 101-year-old angler, it was getting fish for his family three times each week. For a 102-year-elderly person, it was holding her small incredible, extraordinary incredible granddaughter (which she said was "like jumping into paradise"); for a 102-year-old karate ace, it was showing hand to hand fighting. Woven together, these straightforward life esteems give intimations concerning what comprises the very embodiment of ikigai: A feeling of purpose, which means and inspiration in life.

The Health Benefits of Ikigai

For quite a long time, specialists have attempted to discover the purposes for a long and healthy life. While the appropriate response is likely a blend of good qualities, diet, and exercise, contemplates having recommended that discovering importance in life is additionally a key segment.

In an investigation, analysts examined information from more than 50,000 members (ages 40 to 79). They found that the individuals who announced having ikigai in their lives had diminished the dangers of cardiovascular sicknesses and lower death rates. Put another way, about 95% of respondents who had ikigai were as yet alive seven years after the underlying study contrasted with the 83% who didn't. It's difficult to tell whether ikigai ensures life span in life through this single investigation; however, the discoveries recommend that having a feeling of purpose can urge one to manufacture an upbeat and dynamic life.

Finding Your Inward Ikigai

There's no single method to discover your ikigai. However, you can begin by posing a couple of necessary inquiries: What satisfies you? What are you acceptable at? What (and who) do you esteem? What spurs you to find a good pace morning? Finding your ikigai will require some investment. The mystery, I regularly tell individuals, is to gain proficiency with the five central pillars of ikigai. Applying the pillars to your life, you can permit your inward ikigai to thrive.

For specific individuals, their Ikigai is copiously clear, and for some, it's a little more subtle. Discovering it can appear to be an outlandish undertaking, yet it's most certainly not! We accept everybody has a purpose. It can merely take a little while to make sense of it. Your Ikigai lies in the focal point of four interconnecting circles of what you love and what you're acceptable at:

- Your energy
- Your mission
- Your calling
- Your livelihood

Ikigai: Four Inquiries to Start Your Act of the Japanese Philosophy on Life Satisfaction

As indicated by Japanese culture, we as a whole have an ikigai, an 'explanation behind being' or a 'way to life satisfaction.' Japan is known for life rehearses that lead to the life span of its kin, arriving at an average life of 83.7 years. Past investigations have demonstrated the Japanese life span to be firmly identified with dietary practices. New examinations on the Japanese way of thinking have demonstrated life satisfaction through ikigai as a crucial part of life span. It appears as though there is a whole other world to life than only food. Ikigai is comprised of four unique subjects. Bit by bit, your own Ikigai will take shape. This is unimaginable immediately and by no means under tension. Regardless, with four inquiries, you as well can begin your excursion to discover your own Ikigai and start your act of the Japanese way of thinking of life satisfaction.

We are Characterizing Ikigai as Training.

Ikigai isn't simply one more guide 'on the most proficient method to be cheerful.' A definitive objective of Ikigai isn't happiness - it's about a life practice towards satisfaction. In the pursuit of happiness, remember that Japan is positioned just 51 on the planet's most joyful nations. Thus ikigai may not be the training for you. Rehearsing your ikigai is characterizing your purpose, your own crucial finding your maximum capacity. The point is to mark what you can best add to the world, the things you're acceptable at, and that give you joy while doing. The individuals who are effectively seeking after practices to find their ikigai have indicated confidence progressively, feeling their essence on the planet is legitimized.

Therapists clarify why recognizing our purpose in life can help us in life fulfillment. They guarantee that If we can discover our ikigai, everything will be simpler and pleasurable. Simple, since we'll exercise our most tuned abilities. Pleasurable because it will appear to merit doing.

Where are Individuals Finding Their Ikigai?

Some individuals feel that they can't discover in their extraordinary capacities or objectives to life satisfaction. Some are ending up living the truth of tormenting themselves up and hauling themselves arduously to work. The sentiment of drive and energy for work has become, however, ancient history. Individuals can regularly think that it's elusive a sparkle for their occupation, and the fantasy about finding their ikigai has not gotten the opportunity to surface.

In a meeting, one companion clarified where his energy aimed at propelling his group to discover life satisfaction originated from. "Years back, it seems that the dearest companion experienced an extended period of anxiety and awful fear every Sunday when thinking about the upcoming weeks' work.

 He was spending such an extensive amount of his life being despondent busy working, and on that, he squandered Sunday night times, fearing the week to come. In the wake of seeing this example that was created, I began to consider what caused him to feel along these lines and how organizations could evade the Sunday evening fear."

At the workplace, one of the first discoveries of inspirational research is that outward inspiration is unachievable; at the end of the day, it is difficult to propel others. At any rate, not to things they are not effectively persuaded to. Researchers call this inherent inspiration. The Japanese way of thinking requests that individuals discover their ikigai characteristically in our past activities. If you think back, you'll recollect as a kid, and you had a characteristic tendency towards something. At the point when adulthood comes, our regular direction is impacted by social-financial variables like; what others are doing, what our folks accept we ought to do, what sort of salary we accept we requirement for specific ways of life.

Four Inquiries to Rediscover Our Specific Direction.

Inundated in the haze of our ordinary, identifying our qualities isn't, in every case, simple. Four inquiries can assist us in finding our way. If you record them in someplace where you go over them routinely, you can utilize them as a compass carrying you closer to your purpose. At whatever point, something new surfaces; simply take a moment to write it down. How about we start.

• What is my component? Do you consider yourself to be an outgoing individual or a thoughtful person? Do you end up enjoying exercises in gatherings or all alone? In some cases, it's a blend, yet make sure to record the sort of organization you enjoy in different circumstances.

• With what exercises do I experience flow? When does your time pass quickly? What is something you could go through hours effectively doing? This is a movement wherein you will feel completely drawn in and won't consider whatever else while doing.

• What do you discover simple to do? Is there anything which you by and by find simple that others appear to battle with? A few people find arranging records in an unmistakable way simple; others are incredible at understanding various perspectives.

• What did you find joyful to do when you were a child? This inquiry builds up the premise of your ikigai. Are your qualities intrapersonal, relational, intelligent, physical (sensation), etymological, aural, or perhaps visual (spatial)?

Ikigai is a Cutting Edge Life.

Ikigai is the association purpose of four significant life segments: enthusiasm, work, calling, and mission. As such, where; what you love meets what you are acceptable at, meets what you can be esteemed, and paid for meets what the world needs. Ikigai is possibly finished if the objective suggests support of the network. We feel more fulfilled by giving blessings than accepting. The subsequent stage, when you've recognized these segments, begins following your compass. Begin taking a shot at your inquiries, and perceive how your answers fit in the Ikigai parts.

The quest for life satisfaction has been a definitive objective of individuals since the very beginning. We look for rehearses that bring us satisfaction, and this is similarly as important all through our time, all things considered in our own lives. The Japanese way of thinking shows that 'ikigai' isn't training to the only delight in outside of work, yet one that ought to be inborn in all parts of our lives.

When it comes to our careers, we will most likely feel dissatisfied if given the burden of waking up each morning only to put superhuman efforts to advance towards a spot where we don't feel esteemed for how we set out excursion with the world. Individuals ought to consistently be a need in any association and, above all, the actualization of their objectives. Even though this may sound gullible, if you deal with the prosperity of your representatives, your outcomes will take off. From a budgetary perspective, putting resources into your group's natural inspiration, your group's ikigai builds your ROI.

These keys are primary and straightforward to try and depend on understanding:

- Do what you excel at
- Know how to state No
- Take care of your vitality
- Practice constant self-improvement
- Stop and choose to accomplish something satisfying.
- Align your qualities with those of your organization
- Simplify, don't make things troublesome
- Love the Why of your organization
- Trust in others

Life Satisfaction and Great Place to Work.

While investigating the possibility of satisfaction in the working environment, one frequently will run over the association, Great Place to Work. This association arrives at the resolution, following a large number of studies and long stretches of broad research, that three significant components need to exist in a decent working environment:

- Trust among associates and leaders.
- Pride in the job you perform.
- Camaraderie in the working environment.

Trust is the primary spot you need to begin; it's the paste to any organization if you need to improve and develop. Trust is subject to the connection between the representative and the organization. It's in the hands of the working environment and group to make upgrades. The aftereffects of acquiring trust in your working environment are incalculable. Representatives are progressively agreeable in their condition, can depend on each other for help, feel esteemed, and are considerably more certain to voice their suppositions and thoughts.

Pride and fellowship are increasingly hard to characterize and acquire. These two qualities are diverse in that they rely upon every distinctive individual, their characters, and their needs. They depend on the connection between the representative and their activity (pride), and the connection between the worker and their colleagues (brotherhood). The requirements every individual must be glad for their activity are close to home and exceptional, and it's significant to guarantee everybody is in a job that fulfills their objectives. The nature of associations with collaborators relies upon the characters and various inclinations every individual has, just as the capacity of the group to coordinate them flawlessly. Pride and fellowship can be connected back to the concept by ikigai when you consider the idea of 'to fall back on toleration when in doubt.' Acknowledging others for their explanation behind being while esteeming yourself as you are, permits a friendly workplace made out of effective people.

Moving to Fulfilling Place to Work

To be an organization made out of satisfied people, you need to initially be an incredible work environment that centers around the three components recorded beforehand; trust, pride, and fellowship. The best approach to turn into a pleasant work environment is very like how you become a satisfied person. You can't concentrate on the satisfaction itself, yet you need to devote yourself to your interests and a balanced lifestyle. It is a procedure explicit to the person just as the working environment. This procedure requires specific instruments, for example, the reality to talk about the four inquiries of ikigai, trust, backing, and clear correspondence.

Saying that you have the most pleasant work environment on

the planet is equivalent to stating you are the most satisfied individual on the planet. This could be valid, yet it's particular and extraordinary to you just; if someone else were from your perspective living your life, they wouldn't feel precisely the same path as you. To be the most satisfying working environment on the planet is dependent on and restrictive to your particular group of people, their purposes behind being, procedures to arrive, and adjust them all. Every worker should be in a job with daily assignments that are lined up with their very own and expert purpose, which brings about the side-effect of life satisfaction. By adjusting individual Ikigais with the work environment objectives, you are following the procedure to make a satisfying association.

The objective of turning into the most pleasant working environment on the planet is one well worth seeking after. If more associations would stop and ask how they could all things considered become a satisfying one, the number of individuals experiencing nervousness and stress would diminish. At the same time, the degree of aggregate satisfaction would unavoidably build objective accomplishment.

What is your Ikigai?

As per the Japanese, everybody has an ikigai. An ikigai is basically 'motivation to find a workable pace morning.' Motivation to enjoy life. Having burned through the greater part of the most recent couple of years, helping handfuls and many business people discover their ikigai while additionally scanning for my own, I would now be able to envision where it has a place.

Your ikigai lies at the focal point of those interconnecting circles. If you are inadequate in one zone, you are passing up your life's latent capacity. That, yet you are passing up your opportunity to carry on with a long and cheerful life. I have made some long memories fixation on anomalies, and curiously enough, some exception networks on the planet live far longer than normal. There are some amazing decisions about the elements that make a long and healthy life. One of the huge variables is ikigai.

Nowadays, my explanation behind getting up is to deal with ventures that rethink society and instruction. For somebody who went through decades battling to discover motivation to get up, it is presently a refreshing change to have this profound feeling of purpose. My health and prosperity have drastically improved during the ongoing years, as well. The essential explanation behind this has not been the healthy options I have made or the diets I have followed, but since I currently live with a feeling of purpose – and that is the stage for the various decisions I make.

The key to a long and cheerful life isn't to live in the expectation of an incredible life tomorrow. It is to live with the aim today. What I love is this is conceivable at the individual level, yet whole networks can gain from it, too.

Have you Discovered your Ikigai?

– Are you accomplishing something that you love?

– That the world needs?

– That you are acceptable at?

– And that you can be paid for?

How might you live with purpose today, to carry on with a longer and healthier life?

The Art of Ikigai

Ikigai is an old eastern way of thinking persistently continuing in Japanese culture. Ikigai essentially implies the explanation behind being. Ikigai is the purpose behind which you get up every morning and for which you live.

The way of thinking of Ikigai is based on these five pillars:

- Starting small
- Releasing yourself
- Harmony and sustainability
- The joy of little things
- Being in the present time and place

Every single one of these pillars coincides in harmony, and together they can improve your life and make it increasingly significant. It usually gives us another view on life, which conflicts with the serious soul pushed onto us by society. You need to accomplish your enormous dreams now, not when you're 60 and biting the dust. I get it; I've felt like that on many occasions.

Yet, consider yourself: Would you be eager to forfeit your health, connections, and the unique moments every day brings to make sure you may become "effective" in a couple of months? The fact of the matter is it's impossible we can realize how tomorrow will unfurl. Our most reliable option is to enjoy today to its fullest and do our best to get it going.

All things being equal, Ikigai is here to spare everybody's day. Before we investigate the five pillars of Ikigai, I need to give you a short case of how wonderful Ikigai is and how it caused individuals to make their progress.

In the spring of 2014, President Barack Obama made his official visit to Japan. The Japanese government was forced because they expected to locate the ideal scene where the Prime Minister could have the welcome supper. Things being what they are, Sukiyabashi Jiro, one of the world's most celebrated sushi eateries, was picked as the scene for the gathering. The café is going by Jiro Ono, who, at the age of ninety-three, is the most established three-Michelin-star gourmet expert. His massive achievement can be credited to his monstrous perseveration yet additionally to his Ikigai. The achievement is certainly not essential for having Ikigai. Achievement can result in a symptom of having ikigai.

Ikigai is available to us all: the cool wind you feel in the first part of the day, the grin you get from clients, the true thankfulness your companions give you; they all speak to ikigai. Coming back to our Japanese café, planning sushi is one of the most multifaceted abilities which require outrageous concentration and persistence. It's artistry in itself, which comprises small, dull, and tedious advances. Envision, he needs to "knead" the octopus for one hour to make it delicate and delicate.

Sushi is his greatest ikigai. Ono once said that he wishes to bite the dust while making sushi. Despite all the enormous battles he has experienced to get ready sushi, he cherishes it. His model is only one of the numerous ways ikigai makes our lives worth living. Be that as it may, recall, your ikigai can, in any event, anything: getting up every morning to see the dawn is ikigai as well.

You may feel that any worth framework you have is just

commendable and legitimized If it converts into substantial accomplishments. This mindset will put anybody under unnecessary tension. We ought to never legitimize our qualities before society. You have unique wants and needs. What is beneficial for me probably won't be helpful for you. Follow your heart and don't let the preferences of society prevent you from living an enjoyable life as per your terms.

Let us investigate the five pillars of ikigai.

1. Starting Small

Starting small and executing each progression with care is the very ethos of this column — and it applies to all that you do in life. High-quality ranchers, for instance, give all their time and exertion into making the best and most delicious produce. They get the dirt right. They prune and water their products with care—their feeling of starting small moves them to go extraordinary lengths.

"It doesn't make a difference how gradually you go as long as you don't stop" — Confucius.

You have enormous dreams, which you know, require extraordinary persistence and tolerance. You wish you could accomplish more in a day. It feels you could've accomplished more that day, isn't that right?

You can rest today realizing you've accomplished all that could be needed, however above all, you've followed your *kodawari*. Japan confronted a fast monetary development after WW2, which permitted the nation to build up the assembling of gadgets and car businesses. Travelers weren't viewed as of extraordinary importance, yet as they needed to confront rivalry from countries like China, Korea, and

Taiwan, it was clear they needed to change their methodology.

Sightseers got one of the primary needs for the Japanese government and of Japan's "Cool" activity, which plans to build the number of voyagers. Numerous sightseers have enjoyed their involvement with Japan and have frequently referenced how high caliber the administrations are. They love the way spotless and clean the nation is, and everything is on schedule. It's critical to comprehend this as it's a case of the Godavari at a large scale level.

It speaks to the pride you take in concentrating on small subtleties. Kodawari likewise implies that you don't need to legitimize your endeavors for any bombastic plans. For instance, Japanese is a nation known for its fixation on developing the "immaculate organic product" Sembikiya is Japan's excellent natural product shop where you can locate the greatest natural products, which come at a significant expense. A Sembikiya muskmelon costs you anything from $200 upwards a piece. It's one of the most profoundly respected leafy foods, even purchased as a blessing.

When you see how much the Godavari went into the creation of such a natural product, the cost doesn't appear to be so high any longer. They treat organic products as a gem, which takes a great deal of time. Individuals with the Godavari aren't happy with "adequate" or "fine and dandy." It hasn't anything to do with hairsplitting but instead pouring your heart into the work you're doing and investing wholeheartedly for every small advance you take. Treat the work you do as though you were the most expert individual on this planet. Do it regularly, cautiously, mindful, and center around achieving the best outcomes you can at the moment.

2. Releasing Oneself

At the point when you discharge yourself, you're ready to relinquish your fixations and see things that issue to you in a more precise and positive light. Rehearsing self-acknowledgment is fundamental to this column — but then, it's likewise one of the most troublesome errands we face in our lives. In any case, If you can beat this hindrance and be content with what your identity is, it very well may be an unbelievably compensating experience.

A youngster doesn't need to worry about the concern of the social meaning of the self, nor is he attached to a societal position yet. It would be so awesome to keep up the way of a joyful kid in life. Releasing oneself is the second mainstay of ikigai and a fundamental piece of the care reasoning which goes connected at the hip with being in the present time and place, the fifth mainstay of ikigai. To all the more likely comprehend the arrival of oneself, we'll accept Zen Buddhism as a commonsense model.

In the suburb of Fukui, Japan, lies the Eihei-Ji sanctuary, which is one of the most durable temples in the nation. It was established in 1244 by Dogen, and it's where it might be clerics learn and train. To be acknowledged as a follower, one must remain for a considerable length of time before the door, regardless of how the climate is. It may be viewed as injurious. However, it is somewhat a procedure of refutation of oneself.

When the follower joins the sanctuary, he won't be dealt with any, not quite the same as the other individual supporters. In such temples, there isn't any legitimacy framework. Regardless of how much work you do, how well you perform, or to what extent you ruminate, you'll get no pats on the head, no acclaim. It could be seen as there would be no material fulfillment at all, nor would you find a good pace inner self.

What you would get is tactile excellence. Every day lived in the sanctuary would be a flow of tangible distinction, which gives you a feeling of endless delight. This happens because you discharge yourself and open to the unbounded universe of tactile joys. Viktor went through 3 years of his life in different death camps. He is driven by a powerful will to live and incredibly good karma; he figured out how to endure the absolute harshest conditions in the world.

They were given continuously something to do under extraordinary climate conditions with scarcely anything to eat and drink. It was only sometimes for them to see anything great by any stretch of the imagination. However, one day, a man drew the consideration of a companion beside him to the unique perspective on the sun setting through the tall trees of the Bavarian woods. It was a dazzling moment as they hadn't seen the magnificence of nature for such a long time. One night when everybody in the camp was lying dead drained in their cabins, one of the detainees came hurrying and requested that everyone amass outside to watch the high dusk.

"Remaining outside, we saw evil mists shining in the west and the entire sky bursting at the seams with billows of ever-changing shapes and hues, from steel blue to dark red. The barren dim mud hovels gave a sharp difference, while the puddles on the sloppy ground dismissed the shining sky.

The absence of any fulfillment from material methods opened another world to the detainees who needed just their opportunities back. You needn't bother with a ton to have significant encounters. Through the arrival of oneself, you can encounter all the more consistently and live every day to its fullest.

Forces outside your ability to control can remove all that you have aside from a certain something, your opportunity to pick how you will react to the circumstance."

3. Harmony and Sustainability

"Sustainability is a specialty of life, requiring inventiveness and ability. A man resembles a woodland, an individual yet associated and reliant on others for development."

You can't accomplish your objectives in case you're continually battling with the individuals around you. Developing — and keeping up — a feeling of the network will furnish you with a robust, emotionally supportive network to help you through life's most testing moments.

The earth where you live will influence you, regardless of how solid your will is. By carrying change to your condition, you'll likewise carry change to yourself. This is the third mainstay of ikigai: harmony and sustainability. Putting our aspirations and wants over everything else can guarantee negative reactions. Your individual wants can be offset by the durability of society and the nature you're living in. Any healthy and hearty community will assist you with accomplishing your objectives and wants. Be that as it may, be careful with not organizing your gain over others.

Harmony and sustainability go connected at the hip with the arrival of oneself. You search externally and endeavor to help other people in making an empowering domain. Don't just do it since it benefits you; however, do it since you can help different citizenry too. In Japan, you'll frequently discover artistic creations of Mt. Fuji on the dividers of the open showers. It's an endeavor to carry nature inside and accomplish harmony with it, even though they live in profoundly urbanized territories.

Japan is a country of sustainability. Their way of life is worked around a mindset which welcomes harmony with nature and among the people of society. You need to think about how every decision you take in a social setting can influence society all in all. You must be accommodating of the individuals impacted by your choice. Along these lines, you can acquire harmony and sustainability in your life, which encapsulates ikigai's type of balance.

A similar mindset can likewise prompt unreasonable pressure and shakiness, both for people and society. Ikigai doesn't welcome a challenge, nor does it welcome a success/lose mindset. As recently referenced, Ikigai is accessible to anybody and can be held under some random conditions.

4. The Joy of Little Things

Discovering joy in the small things — the morning air, some espresso, or the beam of daylight — ought to be a piece of what propels you to find a good pace. In secondary school, I would take the equivalent 6:20 a.m. train to class each day. The sight of a similar recognizable appearance enjoying a round of *shogi* (Japanese chess) consistently gave me enormous joy.

Karoshi is a word that has been Included in the global dictionary. It signifies "passing from the exhaust." Japan is known to be a nation whose individuals follow an exacting hard-working attitude, which, as a general rule, consumes them out and prompts negative causes. It has gotten dominant in Japanese society. To counter-assault it, individuals have begun to follow pastimes. Numerous Japanese representatives are not satisfied with their work, and they search for an approach to adjust their work and individual lives.

Ikigai can bring a feeling of fulfillment through the joy of small things wherein one will enjoy a leisure activity in a significant manner. You get a tremendous sense of accomplishment after seeing through with an undertaking. "Fulfillment originates from making something through and through, where individuals appreciate both the procedure and the outcome." It is critical to comprehend that you may have a 9 to 5 employment and still be cheerful as long as you find the workable pace you need.

Consistently it ought to be your plan to do in any event one thing you need to. This carries happiness and satisfaction to you and makes every day worth living. The joy of little things goes connected at the hip with starting small. Whatever your diversion may be, it doesn't need to something pretentious. It very well may be anything: eating vegetables you developed in your home nursery, welcoming clients with a grin, composing short stories.

You are not bound somewhere around any models. You are allowed to do anything you desire, regardless of how inconsequential it might appear to other people. You are doing it since you follow your heart. The millennial business people have caused individuals to accept they must be fruitful simply like them, so their activities can be defended and merit something. Do what you see fit. No one but you can choose what is positive or negative for you. Pick something, start small, and invest wholeheartedly in every single step you take towards overseeing the undertaking.

5. Being in the Present Time and Place

This column is maybe the most significant. To be in the present time and place, it's imperative to concentrate on the present and practice care each day. Numerous sumo grapplers affirm that being in the current time and place is entirely fundamental in getting ready for and battling in a session. They guarantee that inundating themselves in the present supports their perspective for ideal execution.

As you saw, every individual column works with each other in delightful harmony. Through the arrival of oneself, you can encounter the being in the present time and place. You'll have the option to live in a persistent condition of euphoria. It will permit you to include an action such a lot of that time passes quickly by. Given the concept of flow, you can discover delight in work. "Work turns into an end in itself, instead of something to be suffered as a method for accomplishing something" This methodology appears to be so nonsensical because we are made to accept we generally need to get something out of our work. If we don't, it adds up to nothing.

Like any person, you are stressed over your government assistance and fulfilling your wants. The arrival of oneself permits you to relinquish your sense of self, which disrupts the general flow of being in the present time and place. "Over and over again, we accomplish something for remunerations. If the prizes are not inevitable, we are baffled and lose intrigue and enthusiasm in work" It's reasonable If you see such an undertaking hard to achieve. It requires some investment to revamp ourselves to another mindset, and it's challenging to do so when you are encompassed by individuals who consistently look for remunerations.

Discovering happiness in one's endeavors is the most significant test in life that you can survive. Compose an article when no one understands it, draw an image when no one is viewing it. Exercise when no one is there to see your improvement—code in any event, when no one will procure you as an engineer. The inward joys you'll get from your work without hoping to get prizes or acknowledgment will be all that could be needed to make you continue with your life.

Find a Sense of Contentment.

"Nobody spares us, however, ourselves. Nobody can, and nobody may. We must walk the way. — Buddha

There is no enchantment recipe for discovering Ikigai. Everybody has an alternate ikigai. You'll need to locate your ikigai through investigation. Since Ikigai requires self-investigation, you have to do one significant thing: acknowledge what your identity is. Figure out how to excuse yourself for whatever you've done or are doing and find a sense of contentment with who you are. In this manner, you'll have the option to make the way towards ikigai. If you need to actualize ikigai in your life, you need to drop your convictions about material achievement and the soul of rivalry.

Possibly you change your convictions or your activities, so you'll forestall intellectual cacophony. Your psyche will be in an incredible interior clash because your actions are not lined up with your convictions or the other way around. When you can adjust yourself intellectually, ikigai will assist you with flourishing regardless of when you are in your life. It will require some investment to become acclimated to ikigai if you have carried on with your life so far, doing the contrary energies of these pillars. You'll feel uneasiness from the outset, yet then it will back out as you construct the establishments of another life on the five pillars of ikigai.

CHAPTER FOUR

THE POWER OF SMALL THINGS OF EVERYDAY LIFE

Energy doesn't originate from significant triumphs or extraordinary accomplishments. Those are rare moments of happiness and fulfillment. If you need to encircle yourself with positive vibrations in regular day-to-day existence, you need to depend on the power of small things. If the day doesn't begin how you need it, you need to condition your psyche to imagine that all is well. The mind resembles a muscle, and the more you train it to support your inspiration, the more it will be responsive to do it again when the following dull day comes.

Eight Tiny Changes to Make Your Life 10-Times More Enjoyable.

I think we are, on the whole, open to making changes in our lives that make us more joyful and increasingly productive. Yet, not many of us finish because focusing on something that is going to change our lives is an overwhelming and enormous endeavor, isn't that so? Not really; rather than concentrating on tremendous, radical advances, begin pushing ahead by consolidating these eight changes that are so small and straightforward that you can execute them right away.

These eight stages can completely change yourself to improve things.

1. Reprogram Your Psyche to Remain Positive.

Our musings and activities are affected by our sentiments. That is the reason when no doubt about it "blah" because the climate is terrible or you had a distressing week, all you need to do is remain in bed. Here's the issue. Antagonism is surrounding us. There's no way around that, either. However, what we can do is figure out how to reprogram our psyches to remain positive. You can't trap each negative idea in the cheerful chappy end zone of your brain. However, you can assume responsibility for your considerations by:

- Keeping a gratitude diary. Scribble down what you're appreciative of consistently as opposed to stressing what you don't have. Gratitude will make you more joyful, increment your profitability, and assist you with resting better around evening time.
- You are creating and rehashing positive confirmations that recognize the advancement you are making in the zones where you need to improve.
- You are surrounding yourself with positive individuals who lift your spirits. Keep in mind; feelings are infectious.
- Don't recognize negative contemplations.
- I am staying dynamic. Exercise discharges endorphins, yet inertness prompts over-dissecting and over-thinking.

2. Set Your Caution 30 Minutes Sooner.

One quality numerous fruitful people share is they find a good pace. While you don't need to wake up at the profane hour of 3:45 a.m. like Apple's Tim Cook, you could begin setting your initial 30 minutes sooner. Along these lines, If you typically set your alert for 7 a.m., set it for 6:30 a.m.

The explanation? This will give you some additional time toward the beginning of the day to exercise, reflect, read, browse your messages, eat with your family, plan your day, or work on something that you're energetic about. It spares you from hurrying out the entryway of every early daytime, feeling absent-minded, unaccomplished and jumbled. The time following is critical to personal development.

3. Tidy up After Yourself Right Away.

To what extent does it truly take to make your bed or wash your morning dishes? Possibly five minutes? Stop and think for a minute. If you don't keep steady over these minor tasks, they rapidly develop. That oat bowl and espresso cup turns into a sink full rank dishes that set aside a ton of effort to clean. Whenever washed promptly, you wouldn't have this cerebral pain.

Also, individuals who quickly tidy up after themselves, such as making their beds each morning, will, in general, be more joyful, just as progressively fruitful since it causes you to feel achieved, evacuates mess, and gives them a feeling of control.

4. Don't Over-Submit.

A typical topic I notice with self-improvement guidance is how individuals make objective setting sound simple. They'll propose that you get more exercise or rest, yet that is more difficult than one might expect when you're working 12 hour days and assisting with an infant. I'm not rationalizing-far from it. If you keep your objectives basic and unmistakably characterized, the process will be finished more effectively. Start small and stir your way up. Try not to bounce into a long-distance race carelessly If you need more exercise. Start with ten push-ups a day, a stroll down your square after supper, or this seven-minute exercise plan that you can do in your room.

If you need to begin eating healthier yet aren't quite a bit of a cook, attempt assistance like Blue Apron or Sun Basket. They send healthy fixings to your home and give you bit by bit directions on the most proficient method to set up the suppers. If you need to begin thinking, start with dedicating five minutes per day. This sounds accurate in the business world too. At the point when we started my organization, we attempted to be everything to everybody. Presently, we center on being the best invoicing organization out there. Don't over-promise and under convey.

5. Try Not to Be so Unsurprising.

Doing every single day likewise places us stuck. Probably the best thing that you can accomplish for yourself is to quit being so unsurprising. Break free out of your range of familiarity in any event once per week and explore new territory that you've never done. Attempt that Thai café. Go snowboarding. Buy a closet from another store.

You get the point. Opening ourselves up to new encounters makes us more joyful, changes our points of view, causes us to perceive new chances, helps vitality, and makes us progressively responsive to change. This cycle hovers back. New encounters will make you more joyful.

6. Swap Griping for Offering Thanks.

In any event, during my darkest occasions, I always attempted to stay hopeful by advising myself that, despite the disappointment of my business, I, despite everything, had the help of my loved ones. Perhaps the ideal approach to feel better when you need it more than anything is by demonstrating your gratitude. Be appreciative of the best thing that transpired today. I previously referenced keeping an everyday gratitude diary, yet I need to pressure this can completely change you. Specialists have discovered that;

- Those who keep a week-by-week gratitude diary will, in general, exercise more, have fewer physical side effects, and are progressively hopeful about their prospects.
- The daily conversation of gratitude can expand readiness, excitement, assurance, mindfulness, vitality, and rest span, also lower reports of misery.
- Individuals who consider, talk about, or expound on gratitude day by day are bound to assist somebody with an individual issue or offer passionate help.
- Those who are appreciative of spotless importance on material merchandise are less jealous of others and are bound to impart their assets to other people.
- Daily gratitude practices may help forestall coronary supply route malady.

Demonstrate your gratitude to your companions, family, customers, and associates. Honestly, expressing gratitude toward individuals is perhaps the most ideal approach to fortify connections. Doesn't it feel magnificent when somebody expresses gratitude toward you for your delicate work, doing an errand, or simply listening when they have to vent?

7. Quit Contrasting Yourself with Others.

Quit losing rest over what others have and what you don't. Here's the reality: there is continually going to be somebody who has a superior paying activity, lives in a more pleasant house, drives a fancier vehicle, and goes on progressively fascinating excursions. Your companions may begin families before you. Some may find a workable pace.

Looking at yourself just makes you hopeless and miserably engrossed about what others think about progress: instead, stress over what you characterize as progress. At the point when I began outsourcing, I had companions who ridiculed me since I wasn't getting as a lot of money as they were. As far as I could tell, I had an adaptable calendar, found a good pace I needed, and never griped about work since I enjoyed what I was doing. My companions that gave me a harsh time whined continually about their employments, associates, getting up so early, and so forth. Who do you believe was more joyful?

8. Handle the One Thing that You've Been Putting Off.

We as a whole put off that specific something: the call to your insurance agency, tidying up your work area, changing the batteries in the smoke cautions. Much the same as those dirty dishes I examined before, setting needs incorporates making certain small errands don't develop until you need to go through a whole day, making up for a lost time. If you have incomplete chores, you are hauling an overwhelming load around with all of you the time, regardless of how small each assignment is. You need to recall it. If conceivable, when you consider it, do it right at that point.

After you've recorded your needs for the afternoon, add a long-standing errand to your plan for the day. For instance, toward the finish of the workday, you'll make that call or compose your working environment since you've just gotten the entirety of your generally significant and vitality depleting errands accomplished for the afternoon. You'll be amazed at how much better and profitable; you'll feel once you've checked these things off your rundown - regardless of whether it's only a psychological rundown.

Free yourself.

Little Things That Can Affect Your Everyday Life Positively.

Those are little disturbances and disappointments of day-by-day life that simply wear on us. Be that as it may, I think the inverse is valid, as well. Small beneficial things can make our daily lives more extravagant and all the more fulfilling. Loads of people as of late got some information about the little things that have a significant effect on their lives. I love this rundown.

- Wake up without caution. The clang of the bell or impact of clock-radio music establishes a bumping pace for your day. Instruct yourself to wake up without warning and simplicity into the day to the sound of the world awakening around you.
- Drink great espresso. Or tea, or chai. Whatever your inclination, blend a quality cup and relish it. You're justified, despite all the trouble.
- The breaking points your drive. A considerable lot of my money related to arranging customers choose to resign to a great extent in light of a crushing trip. If you can't live nearer to work, check whether you can get a strategic scheduling plan that permits you to miss heavy

traffic.

- Wear agreeable shoes. No garment has such a significant amount of power over us. Awkward shoes can destroy your day. Indeed, this is an intense one for ladies; however, they attempt to find some kind of harmony between design and solace when purchasing work shoes.

- Be agreeable in your work area. Ensure your seat offers the correct help and that your PC screen is set and upgraded to diminish eye fatigue. Think about a high-quality work area.

- Move around. The benefits of even restricted day-by-day physical movement are about unending. Stroll to your lunch arrangement. Take the canines for a walk this evening. Take a dip each Saturday. Some change is superior to none, and it will cause you to feel better.

- Keep your home clean and composed. This is an ensured pressure reducer, as it makes every errand – from finding a book to preparing for work — slightly simpler.

- Eat great food. It doesn't need to be extravagant, privately sourced, or natural. Be that as it may, the more straightforward and fresher, the better.

- Rest on great sheets. Rest is fundamental to our health and happiness. Try not to let modest, scratchy clothes keep you conscious around evening time.

- Comprehend your impact. You - and just you — have the power to improve everything without exception in your life. Try not to grumble. Fix it. Try not to like your activity? Work to promote it or get another one. Try not to like how the business assistant addressed you? Address it. Discontent with your nearby government? Get included. Need to be better at golf? Take the exercises.

- Be appreciative. We live in a stunning time, and you likely live superior to 99% of the people who have strolled this Earth, including rulers and sovereigns. Recollect that when you are going to get all worked up over what is, in actuality, a small burden.

Small Things Can Help You Get Through The Day With Ease

Small things are powerful. An essential grin, melody, or smell can turn a whole day around. Little things lift you, in any event, for 60 minutes and cause life to appear to be uncommon and justified, despite all the trouble. That is the power of small things. Beneath, you'll discover 20 little things which will make you grin, snicker and put a touch of sparkle in your day.

1. Change your sheets. There is nothing very like the sentiment of clean sheets. It very well may be an agony to strip your bed and put new sheets on, yet the feeling of staying in bed with clean sheets far exceeds the push to put them on!
2. Smell something exquisite. It's been demonstrated that smelling decent things, similar to flowers, a most loved fragrance, prepared treats, or even espresso, has the power to lift our state of mind. So overdo it on a $5 pack of flowers for yourself, splash on some aroma and enjoy the lift it gives you.
3. Get out in the sun. Science has demonstrated that 10

minutes of daylight daily has the power to enact feel-good synthetic substances in your body. So proceed to hang out in the sun and let it warm you awake for ten minutes.

4. Turn your living room into a cinema. Bring a little piece of the film understanding into your home by transforming your living room into a theater. Get some film banners for the dividers, have a 'treat stand,' and enjoy some incredible evenings in. For motivation, look at this present lady's living room change – it's truly noteworthy.

5. Find a moment of wonder. The natural world is loaded with amazement. Stroll to the topmost point of a slope, head to the seashore at dusk, or investigate the detail of a flower. Simply go through five minutes being awed ordinarily.

6. Gratitude. The way today by day gratitude is to fit it into your regular daily existence. It might be that at supper with your family, you each express two things you're thankful for, or when you first stroll through the entryway when you return home from work, you put your keys down and put in almost no time considering three things you are appreciative for. Whatever works for you, simply make it an everyday custom.

7. Eat unique. Pick an organic product or a vegetable from the grocery store that you don't perceive and proceed to make a feast out of it.

8. Do something for another person. Making somebody a pleasant supper or keeping in touch with them a transcribed note mentioning to them what they intend to, you won't just light up their day, however yours also.

9. Take pictures. Snatch your telephone or your

camera, prepare lunch and head out into nature and begin snapping photographs of things that take your extravagant or that make you grin. Search for decent bits of design, the development of grass, or a beautiful cloud arrangement. You will be astonished by all the things you miss or avoid past in your everyday life. Motivation is out there; proceed to look for it!

10. Get some culture. As indicated by examines, visiting an exhibition hall, craftsmanship display, theater, or joining a neighborhood club can help happiness levels and lower tension and wretchedness.

11. Call somebody consistently. Talking to those we like and love can truly get us out of our heads and go into life. You don't need to discuss war and harmony; a straightforward ten-moment 'How's things?' can have a significant effect on your day.

12. Learn another aptitude. There are lots of exercises on YouTube, just like online courses. If you need to get another ability, it's as simple as turning on the PC. Think about all the beautiful things you could get the hang of drawing, sewing, dialects, cooking, fencing, how to support your vehicle... the rundown continues forever!

13. Chocolate treat. Do you like hot cocoa? Why not attempt the most depraved form ever! Just purchase a square of chocolate, dissolve it down, include some warm milk, and mix. Euphoria!

14. Do what you adored as a youngster. Did you love flying a kite? Rounds of Monopoly? Making figures out of the earth? Go through an hour or so doing a movement that you used to cherish as a child and feel your joy levels take off.

15. Add an eruption of shading. Shading has the power

to influence our state of mind. Why not include a splendid burst into your life with a layer of brilliant nail clean, or a bright cup for your morning espresso, or even a beautiful pack of modest and lively flowers for your bedside table.

16. Ask a fundamental inquiry on Facebook. "What was the most entertaining thing you have seen today?" Or you could attempt "What is the kindest thing you have seen today?" the varieties are interminable. However, the outcome will be a rundown of natural goodness to reestablish your confidence in individuals!

17. Hug somebody. At the point when individuals embrace, synthetic concoctions are discharged in their minds, which causes them to feel great. Free Hugs development has the correct thought!

18. Smile and chuckle. Indeed, it may appear as though the exact opposite thing you need to do, however splitting a major wide grin as you mean it, for ten entire seconds, can improve your state of mind.

19. Buy a present for another person. Strangely, examines have demonstrated that we get more delight out of giving a blessing than getting one. So If you need a shot in the arm, head to the shops, pick a little something for someone, wrap it, and part with it. At that point, ride the feelgood vibe for the following barely any hours.

20. Get Happy. Glad is the most joyful tune on the planet. So in case you're battling, fly on Happy and have a move.

CHAPTER FIVE

THE FLOWS OF IKIGAI

Much research shows the stuff to satisfy us, humans. The expression "flow" is utilized to portray how individuals feel when they are entirely occupied with or in "the zone" with what they are doing. Individuals are retained to such an extent that time never appears again to exist. They neglect to eat, drink, and even rest—the necessary conditions for individuals to get into the flow and, consequently, happiness. Happiness can be accomplished through flow autonomous of one's outer states.

To get into the flow, initially, individuals need to see a clear objective and know about directions or rules on how to approach accomplishing the goal. Furthermore, they should see to have the fitting aptitude to execute the regulations or instructions, just as, get immediate criticism on their advancement towards the objective. Thirdly, individuals must have the option to focus and spotlight on the execution and the input they get during the performance.

I wanted to see the similitude between this "Human Flow" and the "Technical Flow" wording utilized in Lean. Technical Flow or a continuous "esteem stream" is the thing that one expects to accomplish in Lean associations. Professional Flow additionally requires unmistakably characterized objectives or Future State. It needs "standard work" or procedure rules, just as a gifted group to progress in the direction of the Future State.

Technical Flow - Human Flow - what different flows would

we say we are mindful of? Indeed, there is the imperative "Cash Flow" that every single business, regardless of how large or small, must be intensely conscious of. Furthermore, significantly progressively famous is the ever-expanding "Data Flow."

Would one be able to incorporate these four flows - Cash, Technical, Information, and Human – into a solitary model? Why not attempt?

I think Cash Flow is the primary flow. Numerous Toyota stories return to the idea that without Cash Flow, one can't be accountable for one's fate. Cash Flow resembles oxygen; all by itself, it has no significance, yet it gives the way to accomplish everything else. Without oxygen, our life finishes as fast as an organization seizes to exist without Cash Flow.

The following flow is Technical Flow. Lean gives a significant number of the standards on the best way to build up and execute flow through the different worth surges of an association. An association, a complex, versatile framework naturally, has sources of info and yields and observes straightforward principles or calculations between its operators. These autonomous specialists inside a sophisticated, versatile structure are human or non-human necessarily.

Specific data sources and yields flow from machine to machine, human to human, human to machine, or a tool to humans. This info and yield flow between the operators establish the Information Flow, which depends on the principles of the Technical Flow. The guidelines of the explicit business game one play. In Lean, for instance, Kaban is an Information Flow framework that alludes to the correct data at the perfect time in the right quality and amount. Lean's "visual administration" framework is additionally part of the Information Flow. Visual administration, similar to a scoreboard in a game, gives input on progress towards an objective or on varieties that alert us to a potential float away from that objective. An Andon is one more noticeable criticism sign of the Information Flow. In synopsis, Information Flow frames the connection or the correspondence channel between the Technical Flow and the Human Flow.

Human Flow, in light of research, is the thing that makes us humans more joyful. To accomplish Human Flow, the accompanying conditions, as talked about, must be met. Individuals need to recognize what to do, the objective, and how to accomplish it, utilizing the standards while having a suitable ability. These conditions are given by the Technical Flow or the Lean framework. The Information Flow provides the proper input required to perceive how one is advancing towards the objective.

The third condition to get into Human Flow, and in this way, a more joyful spot is the capacity to focus on the job that needs to be done. I at first battled with this bright condition. I currently think this the fundamental purpose behind the concept of waste or "*muda*" in Toyota's reasoning. Squander meddles with the flow. Squander diverts us from our capacity to think. The word reference meaning of a "concentrate" is a "substance made by expelling or decreasing the weakening specialist; a concentrated type of something." In Lean, this likens to "esteem include" just, no irrelevant material, work, transport, or and so on. As it were, we expel squander from our frameworks so we can entirely focus on the real job that needs to be done. The errand that drives legitimately to the ideal objective with no temporary re-routes.

Ozgene's vision "to propel humanity" can accordingly be interpreted as "to expand happiness" in light of the Human Flow concept. Ozgene's image to "rouse interest" depicts the individual assessing if the test and saw ability are fittingly adjusted. If the parity is correct, an individual will get inquisitive. If the objective is set too high, more preparation is required, or the individual will get on edge. If the test is unreasonably low for the given aptitude level, the individual will become exhausted rapidly and necessities a higher analysis.

The purpose of the Lean framework, the Technical Flow, is consequently to permit humans to get into Human Flow and henceforth more happy staff. The yield of the Technical Flow makes for glad customers by limiting lead times, seeking after zero deformities, and limiting expenses. Pleased customers settle Cash Flow. Thus the temperate cycle keeps on flowing.

The entirety of this Technical Flow and happiness sound too implausible? Watch individuals play computer games on their cell phones. Clear objectives, clear principles, moment criticism, and all-out focus - they lose all feeling of time - and in any event, until further notice, they are in the zone and feel glad.

Ikigai, Flow, and Longevity

In a period of urban pressure and web-based life interruption, Ikigai reveals insight into the importance of the center, social ties, a healthy lifestyle, and a more prominent feeling of purpose. Japan is known for its commitment to disciplines, going from the structure and car assembling to information the board and culinary specialty. Okinawa islanders can likewise show us a great deal about life span. Various examinations have concentrated on the lifestyles of centenarians from Okinawa and other 'Blue Zones' of the reality where individuals live the longest, for example, Sardinia, Loma Linda, Nicoya, and Ikaria. They also experience the ill effects of less constant sicknesses and enjoy elevated levels of essentialness.

1. Ikigai

Ikgai converts into "the happiness of continually being occupied." As appeared in the Venn diagram over, this "existential fuel" lies at the crossing point of what you love, what you are acceptable at, what you can be paid for, and what the world needs. It is one of a kind for everybody and can change throughout life. In that sense, ikigai is considerably more than energy or calling. This system would make for an extraordinary conversation on subjects like social business, and it would have been valuable for the creators to incorporate such an examination. If one has a feeling of purpose in life, the concept of retirement doesn't make a difference.

It draws on the investigation into logotherapy (finding purpose), which centers around the future, otherworldliness, and reframing current settings. Points of view can be reset by looking at the present from a future state and standing out the contemporary setting from most pessimistic scenario situations. It is imperative to acknowledge sentiments of tension, fear, or stress; in any case, one ought not to capitulate to them or even attempt to dispense with them.

2. Mindset

Individuals who live the longest have a positive disposition and a high level of passionate mindfulness. They can deal with their feelings during times of misfortunes. Reflection "hinders the rotator" of the brain. Care builds true serenity and acknowledges the more significant, just as the better parts of life. While a low degree of weight and infrequent pressure might be gainful, constant pressure is physically unsafe and can cause weariness, discouragement, fractiousness, sleep deprivation, and nervousness.

A solid comical inclination and grinning at individuals (even outsiders) help too. Aloofness helps control interruptions of delight and want through equalization as opposed to disposal. A solid feeling of resilience conquers obstacles and be adaptable to adjust and switch strategies. "Hostile to delicacy" can be worked by making redundancies (e.g., numerous income streams, fellowships outside connections), spreading wagers, and lessening delicacy (e.g., maintaining a strategic distance from harmful individuals, decreasing computerized interruption).

3. The Flow

The concept of flow is characterized as "the state wherein individuals are so associated with a movement that nothing else appears to issue; the experience itself is charming to such an extent that individuals will do it at the extraordinary expense, for the sheer purpose of doing it." An adequate degree of challenge continues the vivid power of flow; an excessive amount of prompts tension, too little prompts fatigue. Making small strides one after another and developing a propensity for discipline moves beyond idleness obstructs into the zone of flow. A stable capacity to center and concentrate is called for to continue flow; unplugging from advanced media ("innovation fasting") helps here. An excessive amount of performing multiple tasks and interference can prompt errors, wastage of time, diminished efficiency, fatigue, sentiment of loss of control, less innovativeness, and powerlessness to recollect what was finished.

It was seen that Japanese experts are eminent for their tirelessness (even fixation) and retention in their assignments, with a careful, tender loving care. "The individuals of Japan have an exceptional ability to make new advancements while saving high-quality traditions and procedures," they clarify. Steve Jobs himself was a major aficionado of Japanese structure in porcelain and gadgets, for example, Craftsman Yukio Shakunaga. The soul of "refined effortlessness" (as opposed to "languid straight-forwardness") is noticeable in Japanese craftsmanship, designing, and food. "The Japanese are gifted at uniting nature and innovation; not man versus nature, yet rather an association of the two," the creators clarify.

It is likewise critical to secure one's existence to bridle ikigai; a specific degree of protection and even isolation is apparent among numerous active individuals. Regular exercises and everyday assignments have a related "microflow" – for instance, Bill Gates says he enjoys washing the dishes around evening time since it unwinds and clears his psyche. Ceremonies additionally have their parts of flow and assist break with bringing down broad objectives into sub-parts.

4. Bits of knowledge from the longest-living individuals

Bits of knowledge are furnished from entrancing meetings with individuals over a hundred years of age, for example,

"Have a colossal hunger for life, I've never eaten meat in my life, I see severely, I hear seriously, and I feel terrible, yet everything's fine"; "Keep your psyche and body occupied" and "I haven't passed on yet." The individuals of Okinawa have a solid feeling of the network and praise the customs of life. It is advised that playing with pets or kids, just as adequate brandishing movement, introduction to the sun, and satisfactory rest.

The conversations with inhabitants of Okinawa share various exercises: invest energy with individuals, sustain companionships, develop a nursery, do the ordinary task, have tea together, slow down, enjoy the little things, be idealistic, accomplish the humanitarian effort, and enjoy chuckling, routine. One likewise should be energetic about what you do, regardless of whether it might appear to be irrelevant, have a purpose or even a few purposes, and praise little things.

5. Food and exercise

An excessive amount of sitting is terrible for muscular and respiratory wellness; ordinary action in small dosages is significant, and this need excludes substantial rec center action. Healthy habits incorporate eating just until the gut is around 80 percent full and eating a differing assortment of vegetables, particularly enemies of oxidants. The "Okinawa diet" includes at any rate five servings of leafy foods every day, of in any event seven sorts.

Everyday things incorporate tofu, miso, harsh melon, ocean growth, soy sprouts, peppers, and green tea. One part covers Eastern controls to unite "body, psyche, and soul, for example, development, stances, and breath in yoga (India), qigong and judo (China), and shiatsu (Japan). On the whole, they gave ten standards refined from their explores are: remain dynamic, don't resign; go slowly; eat healthily; encircle yourself with companions; get fit as a fiddle; grin; associate with nature; allow gratitude every day; live at the time, and follow your ikigai.

Finding a 'Flow' in All that You Do

Looking carefully, Ikigai is "care." I unequivocally accept that Ikigai and care (being at the time) are firmly related in their methodology and offer a lot of standards. Both frameworks need to discover flow in all that you do. Do what you like to an ever-increasing extent, and delayed down when you do what you won't — don't do it in a rush. Your Ikigai is in each one of those small things which you like to do each day.

There is an intriguing concept of "Microflow, enjoying commonplace errands." We've known about probably the best individuals on the planet rehearsing microflow. Bill Gates has been said to wash dishes each night. He professes to enjoy it entirely since it encourages him to unwind and clear his psyche. He even attempts to improve every day – following a full request of his creation, similar to plates go first, forks come next, glasses last. These are his everyday moments of 'microflow.' This is like "being at the time," wherein even daily errands like washing dishes, clothing, cutting flowers, or work area work appear to be enjoyable.

Neuroscientists are diving into "what happens to the cerebrum when we are in that condition of flow?" Up until now, they've found that when we are careful, we are exceptionally perceptive, with determined concentration and no interruptions. Therefore, imagination, efficiency, and happiness develop. The inverse happens when you end up losing the center while working around something you think about significant.

Seven procedures to support your odds of accomplishing flow

1. Comprehending what to do
2. Realizing how to do it
3. Realizing how well you are getting along
4. Realizing where to go
5. Seeing critical difficulties
6. Seeing noteworthy abilities
7. Being liberated from interruption

Much like muscles and the mind, "the more you train, the more you get into the flow," and the closer you find a workable pace.

Ikigai: The Ideal Harmony Among Purpose and Enthusiasm

Finding your own Ikigai is tied in with "focusing" on what makes your inward cognizant self-move. An intriguing component to accomplish this ideal parity is how to transform work and available time into spaces for development," Garcia says. If you need to carry on with long and upbeat life, there must be an Ikigai in your sights, a purpose that guides you for the duration of your life, pushing you to make things of excellence and utility for the network and yourself.

The ten standards of Ikigai, considered through long stretches of research:

1. Continuously stay dynamic: Purpose is critical for

remaining dynamic in life. Individuals who lose enthusiasm for things likewise lose purpose in life. So don't abandon things you love to do both in close to home or expert life.

2. Go moderate: In a meeting, I talked about a 'rushed disorder ' that our reality is confronting. The more significant part of us don't have time; we eat quickly, talk quickly, need results quickly, our capacity to focus has gotten so little, and we need data fast. This is the specific explanation behind our pressure and early burnout. To accomplish Ikigai – go moderate.

3. Try not to fill your stomach: When we eat food, stretch receptors in the stomach are initiated. The Vagus nerve interfaces our stomach, and the cerebrum sends these signs as our stomach fills. It takes around 10 to 20 minutes for the mind to get a succession of correspondence from stomach-related hormones discharged by the gastrointestinal tract (our gut). At the point when you understand that your stomach is 80 percent full while eating, it is generally the worthy furthest reaches of your stomach. Additionally, when you chew gradually, you permit time for this correspondence.

4. Encircle yourself with old buddies: Connect with your old companions, find new fellowships. Spend probably some piece of your day with your old buddies. Companions keep your energies alive and bolster you during your time.

5. Get fit as a fiddle: When you are suitable as a fiddle, your certainty improves. Even though looks are positively not all that matters, a great shape develops self-assurance and subsequently assists you with looking and feel vastly improved. From sparkle on your skin, the sparkle in your hair to entire body

shape, pretty much every part of your body can improve when you're fit as a fiddle

6. Grin: A real grin cause you to appear to be progressively appealing, agreeable, and even trustworthy. Science has additionally demonstrated that grinning makes you healthier, and you will, in general, live longer. There are uncountable benefits like it improves the state of mind, brings down your circulatory strain, discharges pressure, betters your safe framework are somewhere in the range of not many to depend on.

7. Reconnect with nature: Keep your telephone in your pocket and enjoy the sights, sounds, scents, and encounters of your environment and particularly nature around you.

8. Express appreciation: Yes, you read it right. Expressing gratefulness improves your health and happiness. Gratitude is the genuine wellspring of youth, health, energy, and life span. Express appreciation to your body, life, friends and family, companions, and million different things to be grateful for.

9. Live at the time, making care: Living at the time permit you to create consciousness of the present experience as opposed to relating or recognizing it with your past encounters, considerations, sentiments, and thus you show signs of improvement in whatever work you have close by.

10. Follow your Ikigai: Once you recognize your Ikigai, figure out how to remain on course and continue following your IKIGAI.

Individuals consistently request to be given "the one key thing" they have to develop care. Like care, "Ikigai" likewise doesn't originate from a solitary practice or worth framework. It originates from experiencing a range of small-scale encounters, none of which fills an intricate need in life without anyone else. In my excursion towards finding out about care and other comparative sciences, I have understood that there is no single unmitigated formula for happiness. Each particular state of life can fill in as the establishment for joy and accomplishment in its ideal manner.

CHAPTER SIX

THE SECRETS OF CENTENARIANS AND SUPERCENTENARIAN PEOPLE FROM OKINAWA: THEIR HABITS AND DIET

Okinawa islands are a sort of "Japanese Hawaii" for their laid-back vibe, seashores, and fantastic climate. Okinawa likewise happens to have one of the most elevated centenarian proportions on the planet: About 6.5 in 10,000 individuals live to 100 (contrast that and 1.73 in 10,000 in the U.S.) Centenarians on Okinawa have survived a ton of change, so their dietary stories are more entangled than a portion of the other Blue Zones. As Buettner composes, numerous healthful Okinawan "food traditions foundered mid-century" as Western impact realized changes in food habits. After 1949, Okinawans started eating less healthy staples like ocean growth, turmeric, and sweet potato, and more rice, milk, and meat.

Okinawans have sustained the act of eating something from the land and the ocean consistently. Among their "top life span foods" are severe melons, tofu, garlic, dark colored rice, green tea, and shitake mushrooms. The quest for the "remedy of youth" has spread over hundreds of years, and the mainland – yet as of late, the chase has fixated on the Okinawa Islands, which stretch over the East China Sea. Not exclusively do the more seasoned occupants enjoy the most extended life hope of anybody on Earth, however most by far of those years are lived in strikingly high health as well.

Of specific note is the quantity of individuals who arrive at 100 years of life. For every 100,000 occupants, Okinawa has around 68 centenarians – on multiple occasions, the numbers found in US populaces of a similar size. Indeed, even by the principles of Japan, Okinawans are lovely, with a 40% more unique possibility of living to 100 than other Japanese individuals. Little marvel researchers have gone through decades attempting to reveal the insider facts of the Okinawans' life span – in both their qualities and their lifestyle. What's more, one of the most energizing components to have as of late got the researchers' consideration is the curiously high proportion of sugars to protein in the Okinawan diet – with a specific abundance of sweet potato as the wellspring of the more significant part of their calories.

It is an incredible inverse of the ebb and flows popular diets that advocate a high protein, low carb diet. Despite the prominence of the Atkins and Paleo diets, in any case, there is insignificant proof that high-protein foods truly achieve extended haul benefits.

So could the "Okinawan Ratio" – 10:1 sugar to protein – rather be the key to a long and healthy life? Even though it would, in any case, be unreasonably right on time to recommend any lifestyle changes dependent on these perceptions, the most recent proof – from human longitudinal investigations and creature preliminaries – propose the speculation is worth genuine consideration. As per these discoveries, a low protein, high sugar diet sets off different physiological reactions that shield us from different age-related sicknesses – including malignant growth, cardiovascular illness, and Alzheimer's sickness. What's more, the Okinawan Ratio may accomplish the ideal dietary equalization to achieve those impacts.

A lot of this exploration originates from the Okinawa Centenarian Study (OCS), which has been researching the health of the maturing populace since 1975. The OCS inspects occupants from over the Okinawa prefecture, which incorporates more than 150 islands. By 2016, the OCS had examined 1,000 centenarians from the area.

Instead of enduring a drawn-out end, the Okinawan centenarians seemed to have deferred a considerable lot of the standard impacts of maturing, with very nearly 66% living autonomously until the age of 97. This astounding "health length" was definite across many age-related infections. The regular Okinawan centenarian gave off an impression of being liberated from the common indications of cardiovascular illness without the development of the hard "calcified" plaques around the supply routes that can prompt cardiovascular breakdown. Okinawa's most established inhabitants likewise have far lower paces of malignant growth, diabetes, and dementia than other maturing populaces.

Hereditary Benefits

Given these outcomes, there is little uncertainty that Okinawa has an extraordinary populace. In any case, what can clarify that different life span?

Hereditary favorable luck could be one significant factor. On account of the topography of the islands, Okinawa's populaces have spent huge lumps of their history in relative disconnection, which may have given them a one-of-a-kind hereditary profile. Starter contemplates proposing this may incorporate a decreased commonness of a quality variation – APOE4 – that seems to build the danger of coronary illness and Alzheimer's. They may likewise be bound to convey a defensive adaptation of the FOXO3 quality engaged with controlling digestion and cell development. These outcomes in a shorter stature yet additionally seem to decrease the danger of different age-related illnesses, including malignant growth.

All things being equal, it appears to be far-fetched that great qualities would completely clarify the Okinawans' life span, and lifestyle variables will likewise be significant. The OCS has discovered that Okinawans are less inclined to smoke than most populaces, and since they worked dominatingly in agribusiness and angling, they were likewise physically dynamic. Their very close networks also help the occupants to keep up a functioning public activity into a mature age. The social association has likewise been appeared to improve health and life span by diminishing the body's pressure reactions to testing occasions. (Dejection, interestingly, has been demonstrated to be as hurtful as smoking 15 cigarettes per day.)

It is the Okinawans' eating routine, in any case, that may have the most potential to change our perspectives on healthy maturing. In contrast to the remainder of Asia, the Okinawan staple isn't rice. However, the sweet potato, first presented in the mid-seventeenth Century through exchange with the Netherlands. Okinawans likewise eat a bounty of green and yellow vegetables –, for example, the unpleasant melon – and different soy items. Even if they do eat pork, fish, and various meats, these are usually a small segment of their general utilization, which is, for the most part, plant-based foods.

The traditional Okinawan diet is in this way thick in the essential nutrients and minerals - including enemies of oxidants - yet additionally low in calories. Especially previously, before cheap food entered the islands, the normal Okinawan ate around 11% fewer calories than the typical suggested utilization for a healthy grown-up.

Therefore, a few researchers accept that Okinawans offer more proof for the life-improving temperances of a "calorie limited" diet. Since the 1930s, a few specialists and researchers have contended that constantly restricting the measure of vitality you devour could have numerous benefits well beyond weight reduction – including a deceleration of the maturing procedure.

In one of the most convincing examinations, a gathering of rhesus macaques eating 30% fewer calories than the average monkey indicated a surprising 63% decrease in passings from age-related sicknesses over a 20-year time frame. They additionally looked more youthful – they had fewer wrinkles, and their hide held its energetic brilliance as opposed to turning dark. Because of useful challenges, long-haul clinical preliminaries in humans still can't seem to be finished to test the consequences for life span. Yet, an ongoing two-year explore, financed by the US National Institute on Aging, was profoundly intriguing: members on a calorie confined eating regimen demonstrated better cardiovascular health – including lower circulatory strain and cholesterol.

It's as yet not clear why a calorie confined eating regimen would be so useful. However, there are numerous potential instruments. One attribute is that the calorie limitation changes the phone's vitality flagging, with the goal to make the body dedicate more assets to conservation and support, as opposed to development and multiplication, all while constraining oxidative pressures brought about by the lethal results of digestion that can cause cell harm.

The Benefits of the Okinawan Diet May Not End with Its Calorie Limitation.

Solon-Biet has led a progression of studies focusing on the impact of dietary creation on maturing creatures. Her group of researchers managed to discover that a high-carb, low-protein diet broadens the lifespan of different species. Her latest examination indicates that said diet lessens a portion of the indications of maturing in mind. Incredibly, they have discovered that the ideal proportion is ten sections carb to one section protein – equivalent to the alleged Okinawan Ratio.

Even though there aren't yet any controlled clinical preliminaries in humans, Solon-Biet refers to epidemiological work over the world that all point to comparable ends. "Other seemingly perpetual populaces have additionally been appeared to have dietary examples that generally incorporate low measures of protein," she says. "These incorporate the Kitavans, [who live on] a small island in Papua New Guinea, the South American Tsimane individuals and populaces that devour the Mediterranean eating routine."

By and by, the specific systems are dim. Like calorie limitation, the low protein diets appear to advance the cell fix and upkeep. Together, these progressions may forestall the maturing related gathering of harmed proteins inside cells. This development of damaged proteins may typically be answerable for some maladies – however, the ordinary tidy-up when we eat a low-protein diet could forestall it.

So would it be right for us to all beginning receiving the Okinawan Diet? Not exactly. Ryan focuses on some proof that low protein admission may restrict, in essence, harm up to the age of 65. However, you may then benefit from expanding your protein consumption after that point. "Ideal nourishment is required to shift over the life history," she says. What's more, it's a likewise significant examination, which found that the overall benefits of protein and starches may rely upon the protein's source. An eating regimen higher in plant-based protein seems, by all accounts, to be superior to an eating regimen wealthy in meat or dairy, for example. So the Okinawans might be living longer because of the way that they are eating (for the most part) products of the soil instead of its high-carb, low-protein content.

Privileged Insights to Living a Longer Life

The most seasoned ladies on Earth possess Okinawa Island. Icaria – an island that is situated in the Aegean Sea – has the enduring populace with the most minimal feeble dementia levels. Loma Linda is home to a network of Seventh-day Adventists whose life anticipation is ten years over the average lifespan in the United States. What's more, in Nicoya, we can locate the second-biggest network of centenarians on the planet.

What is the mystery behind this extraordinary life span, the riddle of the blue zones, where such a significant number of centenarians live?

A group made out of a few authorities (specialists, anthropologists, demographers, nutritionists, disease transmission experts) – ventured out commonly to the distinctive blue zones. They distinguished the accompanying nine general life span factors, which are identified with diet and lifestyle:

    1. Intense and regular physical activity in the

exhibition of daily obligations. The concept of an inactive lifestyle is obscure to the individuals living in these locales

2. Having an "ikigai" – a Japanese word (Okinawa) which is utilized to characterize our own "explanations behind being" or, all the more unequivocally, the reasons why we get up each morning

3. Reduction of stress – a factor which is firmly connected to practically all maturing related maladies. Stress decrease implies intruding on the typical pace of our everyday lives to permit time for different exercises, which are a piece of ordinary social habits—for instance, sleeping in Mediterranean social orders, asking on account of Adventists, the tea service of ladies in Okinawa, etc.

4. "Hara Hachi Bu" – a Confucian training that implies we ought not to keep on eating until we are full, however just until 80% of our eating limit

5. Prioritizing an eating regimen that is wealthy in plant-based items. Meat, fish, and dairy items might be expended, yet in lower sums

6. A moderate utilization of mixed refreshments, which affirms the conviction that reasonable consumers live longer lives than nondrinkers

7. Engaging in social gatherings that advance healthy habits

8. Engaging in strict networks with standard strict practices

9. Building and keeping up secure connections between relatives: guardians, kin, grandparents, and others.

To summarize, the over nine life span variables could be integrated into only two.

Initially, keeping up a healthy lifestyle – which infers customary force exercise, including schedules to "break" from day by day stress, and including fundamentally plant-based items in our diets, gobbling without topping off and not drinking too much.

Furthermore, coordinating in bunches that advance and backing those "great practices": family, strict networks, social gatherings, etc. – all of which must have their own "ikigai," that is, their personal "motivation to live." There is an individual "ikigai," yet there is likewise a group "ikigai" that defines the objectives for every network just as the difficulties in defeating to accomplish them.

Living along these lines implies living better and longer. Hereditary qualities might dictate life span. However, it is additionally something that can be prepared, as can be found in the case of the occupants of the blue zones.

CHAPTER SEVEN

TRADITIONS AND PROVERBS FOR HAPPINESS AND LONGEVITY

Happiness and Longevity - Deities of Good Fortune in Japan

In Edo-period Japan (1603-1868), long and upbeat life was accepted to be the endowment of a gathering of good divinities known as the Seven Gods of Good Fortune (Shichifukujin). This sacred get-together of arranged deities joined four Buddhist causes: Bishamonten, Daikokuten, Benzaiten, and Hotei; two got from the Daoist tradition: Fukurokuju and Jurojin; and one obtained from Shinto conviction: Ebisu. To get benefits from these divine forces of karma, individuals made yearly visits to the sanctuaries committed to their love. Depicting the divine beings filled a similar need; in this manner, they turned into an essential topic in the ukiyo-e woodblock printing tradition, the significant artistic expression of the Edo time frame. At first, portrayals of these gods were treated as consecrated pictures. After some time, such prints developed into frequently funny sort pictures. Numerous such photos were delivered available to be purchased during the New Year.

An exceptional appearance does not recognize the creatures portrayed in progress on seeing. Neither stately nor grave, regularly described by offbeat highlights and conduct, they grin affably and look agreeable, as befits mainstream divinities who bring happiness and thriving. This show grasps a time of more than 180 years—from early tests with shading woodblock prints up to the finish of their history as outstanding workmanship. Planned by Harunobu, Toyoharu, Shigemasa, Hokusai, Gakutei, and others, these prints happen in an assortment of organizations, including tight, upstanding "column prints" (Nashira-e), enormous size print boards (ōban), secretly appointed and distributed grand prints (surimono), sketchbooks (manga), and collections. The divinities show up in their traditional appearance and in comic/ridiculed structures (imitate) as kids or mistresses.

Also, well-known Japanese religion embraced the Chinese faction of built-up Daoist gods known as *sennin*, frequently alluded to as "Immortals." Usually professed to be recorded figures, sending are said to have acquired the mystery of everlasting life, in this way setting a promising model as perfect creatures. Among the Japanese lords of favorable luck, Fukurokuju and Jurōjin are related to life span through their Daoist source.

The assortment of visual understandings for these seven personages isn't unusual: the immortal human mission for happiness and life span started craftsman's minds. We keep on longing for the liberal blessings of the Gods of Good Fortune and just expectation that technological advancement will make them much increasingly productive. The twentieth-century print by Raifu shows a fortune pontoon impelled by steam.

Moai—This Tradition is Why Okinawan People Live Longer, Better

Seniors in Okinawa, Japan, one of the first blue zones life span hotspots, live exceptionally preferred and longer lives over nearly any other person on the planet. Moai, one of their life span traditions, are social care groups that start in adolescence and reach out into the 100s. The term started several years back as a method for a town's money-related emotionally supportive network. Initially, movies were shaped to pool the assets of a whole city for ventures or open works. If an individual required funding to purchase land or deal with a crisis, the main path was to pool cash locally. Today the thought has extended to turn out to be to a higher degree a social, encouraging group of people, a social tradition for worked in friendship.

In small neighborhoods across Okinawa, companions "meet for a typical purpose" (some of the time days by day and in some cases a few days every week) to chatter, experience life, and to share counsel and even budgetary help when required. They consider these gatherings their moai. Traditionally, gatherings of around five little youngsters were matched together, and it's then that they made a promise to one another forever. As their subsequent family, they would meet consistently with their moai for both work and play and to pool assets. Some movies have kept going for more than 90 years!

One of the ladies and blue zones scientists had the delight of meeting in Okinawa was Klazuko Manna, who, at 77 years of age, was the most youthful of her moai (aggregate age of the gathering was more than 450!). She focused on that it isn't just about tattle and jabber — it's profound help and regard for one another. "Every part realizes that her companions depend on her as much as she relies on her companions. If you become ill or a companion passes on or If you come up short on cash, we realize somebody will step in and help. It's a lot simpler to experience life, knowing there is a security net." Even today, about a portion of Okinawans take part in a moai, and many are in more than one.

During the examination and investigations on Okinawa, they addressed many Okinawan nonagenarians and centenarians about the job of moai in their life. He invested energy with Gozei Shinzata, who was as yet spry, lively, and cooked and planted day by day at 104 years of age. He depicts her everyday schedule in The Blue Zones Solution: In the cool hours of the day, she worked in her nurseries. At lunch, she blended handcrafted miso into a pot of water. She spooned in new carrots, radishes, shiitake mushrooms, and tofu and let it heat. In the interim, she went here and there the kitchen cleaning off the counters, sink, and even the window. At the point when it was prepared, she emptied her warmed soup into a bowl, checked it for a few seconds, and mumbled, "Hara Hachi bu." This Confucian proverb, articulated like a petition before each supper, reminded her to quit eating when she was 80 percent full.

After lunch, she read comic books or viewed a ball game on TV and snoozed. Neighbors halted by each evening, and a few days every week, her moai — four ladies who, together with Shinzato, had at a young age focused on each other forever — made a trip for mugwort tea and discussion. At whatever point things had gotten unpleasant in Shinzato's life, when she'd run low on cash or when her better half had kicked the bucket 46 years prior, she'd relied on her moai and the Okinawan feeling of social commitment — *yuimaru* — to help her. Her companions had depended on a lifetime of Shinzato's help consequently.

One examination investigated the association between marital status, ties with companions and family members, club enrollment, level of volunteerism, and a more prominent life span. The examination found that the kind of association was insignificant. Regardless of whether it was a spousal relationship or a very close companion gathering, all that made a difference was the bond the group shared.

Research shows that your social associations can have long-haul sway on your health and happiness. You imitate the habits of your three dearest companions. If you share comparable qualities, healthy habits, and life objectives, at that point, you're probably going to:

1. Experience less Stress

Forlornness can diminish your life hope by eight years. In Okinawa, individuals from a moai experience the pressure, shedding security of realizing that there is consistently somebody there for them.

2. Be Happier

With each upbeat companion you add to your system, you increment your happiness by 15 percent. Happiness is infectious.

3. Live Longer

More seasoned individuals without dear companions are bound to create persistent illnesses, for example, coronary disease, diabetes, and despair, than their partners. They're additionally at a higher hazard for experiencing a stroke.

By and large, they live eight years longer than American ladies. Their moai is likely a significant part of their long lives. In each of the five blue zones societies, social connectedness is imbued into the way of life. While Okinawans have Moais, Sardinians meet with companions each night for glad hours, and Adventists have week-by-week dinners with their assemblies. By finding the correct clan, you'll add a very long time to your life. However, you'll enjoy your time here only a little more.

Happiness Proverbs from all Over the World

If it doesn't execute you, it will bring you happiness. ~ Native American Proverb

Where there is love, there is happiness. ~ Polish Proverb

Happiness has its underlying foundations — distress has its belly. ~ Chinese Proverb

Genuine happiness comprises in satisfying others. ~ Hindu Proverbs

One moment of extraordinary happiness drags our life by a thousand years. ~ Japanese Proverb

Happiness itself doesn't remain — just moments of happiness do. ~ Spanish Proverb

Who tidies up the earth washes away happiness. ~ Mongolian Proverbs

For a few of us, happiness comes while we rest. ~ French Proverb

The happiness that keeps going too long crown jewels the heart. ~ Italian Proverb

Today all around lived makes each yesterday a fantasy of happiness, and each tomorrow a dream of expectation. Look well, along these lines, right up 'til the present time. ~ Indian Proverb

Happiness resembles precious stone — when it sparkles the most, it before long splits. ~ Turkish Proverb

If you need happiness for 60 minutes — sleep, if you need happiness for a day — go angling. If you need happiness for a month — get hitched. If you need happiness for a year — acquire a fortune. If you need happiness for a lifetime — help another person. ~ Chinese Proverb

To have the option to revile once a day improves happiness and stretches life. ~ Chinese Proverb

The happiness in your pocket, don't spend everything. ~ Chinese Proverb

Happiness spring — cleans the heart. ~ Japanese Proverb

Happiness resembles a sunbeam, which the least shadow captures, while misfortune is frequently as the downpour of spring. ~ Chinese Proverb

The burden is he who professes to have discovered happiness. ~ Iranian Proverbs

Happiness takes off from the individuals who need it most. ~ Laotian Proverb

The individual who stalls out on frivolous happiness won't achieve incredible happiness. ~ Tibetan Proverb

There is no winter without a day off, spring without daylight, and no happiness without partners. ~ Korean Proverb

Happiness seldom keeps the organization with an unfilled stomach. ~ Japanese Proverb

Preferable an ounce of happiness over a pound of gold. ~ Yiddish Proverb

Quiet is the mediator of happiness. ~ Arabian Proverb

Happiness opens the arms and shuts the eyes. ~ German Proverbs

At the point when aspiration closes, happiness starts. ~ Hungarian Proverbs

While we seek happiness, we escape from satisfaction. ~ Hasidic Proverb

Yesterday is nevertheless a fantasy, tomorrow yet a dream. In any case, today, all around lived makes each yesterday a fantasy of happiness, and each tomorrow a dream of expectation. Look well, along these lines, right up 'til the present time. ~ Indian Proverbs

Whoever doesn't regard certainty will never discover happiness in their way. ~ Traditional Proverb

Happiness and glass break, no problem at all. ~ Danish Proverb

Happiness isn't a pony; you can't saddle it. ~ Russian Proverbs

Happiness doesn't originate from happiness itself, however, from the excursion towards accomplishing it. ~ Finnish Proverbs

Nobody is more joyful than he who has confidence in his happiness. ~ German Proverbs

God is a dad; happiness is a stepfather. ~ Yiddish Proverb

Happiness doesn't give; it just loans. ~ Danish Proverbs

An expanded thought can blast the air pocket of your happiness. ~ Myanmar Proverb

With happiness comes insight into the heart. ~ Chinese Proverb

There is no different happiness yet harmony. ~ Thai Proverb

Quotes on Longevity

Life span right now about having the option to reevaluate yourself or concoct the future - Satya Nadella

Life span is the way to progress - Ed Seykota.

To accomplish the life span, you will have cycles. Nobody arrives in one straight shot - Rob Lowe.

Long life is a life very much spent - Leonardo da Vinci.

How would you carry on with long life? Go for a two-mile stroll each morning before breakfast - Harry S. Truman.

There can be a ton of life span in the reiteration of things being told again and again in an assortment of ways - Kate Dicamillo.

It's an excellent exciting ride in case you're fortunate to have a life span right now must have the option to ride those waves - Jennifer Lopez.

A long life may not be sufficient. However, a decent life is sufficiently long - Benjamin Franklin

A comical inclination has been connected with life span. It is a likelihood that the psychological disposition reflected in an energetic comical inclination is a significant factor inclining a few people toward long life - Raymond Moody.

The way to fantastic health and life span is to eat a high proportion of micronutrients to macronutrients - Joel Fuhrman.

The mystery of long life is dual vocations. One to about age sixty, at that point another for the following thirty years - David Ogilvy

An unimportant life span is something beneficial for the individuals who watch Life from the sidelines. For the individuals who play the game, an hour might be a year, a solitary day's worth of effort an accomplishment forever - Helen Hayes.

The key to life span is to continue breathing - Sophie Tucker

There is just a single difference between a long life and a decent supper: that, in the supper, the desserts come last - Robert Louis Stevenson

Being proficient is simply actually plainly the best approach and causes you to make a course for life span - Amanda Seyfried.

Long life is a weight when it's spent in wretchedness - Laini Taylor

The man who has experienced the longest isn't he who has

spent the best number of years, yet he who has had the best reasonableness of life - Jean-Baptiste Rousseau.

There's a long life in front of you, and it will be wonderful, as long as you continue cherishing and embracing one another - Yoko Ono.

Long-life will some of the time cloud the star of acclaim - Marie de Rabutin-Chantal.

Everyone is an excellent human being, and we're fortunate. That is the thing that gives you a life span. You need to cherish the individuals that you work with - Katee Sackhoff

The life span of progress relies upon how well you deal with your leaps forward - Constance Chuks Friday.

A human being would not develop to be seventy or eighty years of age if this life span had no importance for the species. The evening of human life should likewise have its very own hugeness and can't be only a desolate member to life's morning - Carl Jung.

We all can hope to live longer than any association that we would work for. That proceeds apace. Human life span is expanding; the corporate life span is diminishing - Dan Pink.

Life span remarkable expansion of the fear of death - Ambrose Bierce

If you need to carry on with a long life, center around making commitments - Hans Selye.

The way to life span is to become familiar with each part of music that you can - Prince.

Positive individuals have more companions, which is a key factor of happiness and life span - Robert D. Putnam.

Life span is a major piece of validity - Jason Calacanis.

The individuals who bite the dust without being overlooked get a life span - Laozi.

The basis for long-living is to remain occupied, get a lot of exercises, and don't drink excessively. Of course, don't drink excessively little - Herman Smith-Johannsen

CHAPTER EIGHT

GENTLE PHYSICAL EXERCISES TO PROMOTE HEALTH AND LONGEVITY

Light Exercise Can Help You Live Longer

An examination shows that small episodes of light physical activity are sufficient to build lifespan in more established men. Government rules suggested that grown-ups get at any rate of 2 hours and 30 minutes of moderate-force exercise each week. Notwithstanding, just about a portion of American adults meet those proposals, and for more established grown-ups, they may appear to be challenging to accomplish. However, another report distributed in the British Journal of Sports Medicine recommends that there's a method to change rules to make them progressively plausible for more seasoned individuals while as yet looking after health.

In the report, scientists took a gander at around 1,180 men — average age, 78 — who consented to wear gadgets that deliberate their developments for seven days. They were followed for about five years. The specialists found that the overall volume of exercise, not really to what extent or how hard somebody exercised in a meeting, made a difference most for life span.

The men in the investigation didn't have to exercise for extensive periods to encounter positive outcomes. Sporadic episodes of exercise for the day, regardless of whether every session was under 10 minutes, had comparable benefits to lifespan as practicing over 10 minutes one after another. This strategy appeared to fit into men's lives, as well; 66% of the men in the examination had the option to meet their week after week prescribed exercise If they did it in shorter blasts.

At regular intervals of light power movement every day — like going on a walk or planting — was connected to a 17% lower danger of early demise in the investigation. Moderate-to-incredible physical action had a significantly more grounded connection to a longer life: doing it was related to a 33% decrease in death hazard for at regular intervals of excrcisc. Nonetheless, the way that light exercise, despite everything, seemed to have a striking life span benefit is significant, the examination writers compose.

If more research can affirm the discoveries, it could propose that getting only a couple of moments of exercise at once — regardless of whether it's light — can bring down the danger of early passing in men. The analysts infer that their discoveries "could refine physical movement rules and make them increasingly reachable for more seasoned grown-ups with low activity levels. They are focusing on the benefits of everything being equal, anyway unobtrusive, from light force upwards," just as urging individuals to do any degree of physical activity for the day.

Exercise for Optimal Health and Longevity

A Lesson from Centenarians

In Okinawa, we heard accounts of anglers who never resign, and I viewed a lady in her nineties hit the dance floor with an enormous jug on her head, something she frequently did. At the point when she wasn't moving, she enjoyed playing traditional Japanese instruments. In Calabria, 110-year-old Salvatore Caruso disclosed to me how he strolled each day to the olive (olive woods) and how much work his olive trees required. In Loma Linda, the exceptionally seemingly perpetual Seventh-day Adventists are celebrated for their significant levels of exercise, including strolling quick and setting off to the rec center.

When Dan Buettner asked exceptionally extensive Costa Ricans to share the key to their life span, they said they enjoyed accomplishing physical work for their entire lives. When I suggested a similar conversation starter to the shepherds of towns with broadly enduring populaces in Sardinia, they disclosed to me that consistently they leave their homes around November, then walk their sheep through bringing down heights and hotter regions, where the creatures can discover food. They don't return until April or May.

What is Physical Movement Best for a Healthy Life Span?

The one you enjoy most, yet additionally the one you can undoubtedly join into your everyday plan and the one you can keep doing up to your hundredth birthday celebration and past. Numerous Okinawans practice hand-to-hand fighting, particularly a move-roused form of jujitsu. The sort of exercise you pick isn't significant. What's notable is working all your body leaves behind meticulousness — which means to the point of breathing quickly or perspiring — for five to ten hours every week.

I'm not looking at running week after week long-distance races. Workaholic behavior in your body is certifiably not a smart thought. If you consider a vehicle, can anyone explain why nobody needs to purchase a 5-year-old vehicle with one hundred thousand miles on the odometer? Despite being moderately new, it has been driven excessively. You can supplant the tires and repaint the undercarriage. However, you can't change each belt, hose, and valve, and there's a high possibility that some worn parts will separate. Then again, you would prefer not to leave your vehicle left in the carport more often than not, as this will likewise in the long run cause it to stall.

Similar remains constant for the human body. It's imperative to exercise, yet not to overexercise, because knees, hips, and joints will, in the long run, get harmed — especially If you keep on practicing when you feel torment. On the bright side, specific exercises and diet can make tissue self-fix and recover, so the human body has worked in preferences over a vehicle.

Step by Step Instructions to Optimize Exercise for Longevity

The accompanying rules are for practicing to amplify health and life span:

Walk quickly for an hour consistently.

The objective of strolling for an hour each day can, without much of a stretch, be accomplished. For instance, pick a bistro or eatery a short way from your work and try going there two times per day. It can likewise be performed toward the end of the week by strolling when you would ordinarily drive. Consistently, I take my USC understudies from Los Angeles to Genoa, Italy, for three weeks. On a principal day, we make a mobile voyage through the city. I, at that point, ask them to keep strolling wherever for the span of the outing. Before the course is finished, they usually spend time walking around the city and have grown to enjoy it, as they feel better when all is said and done.

Run, Ride, or Swim about Forty Minutes Each other Day, in Addition to Two Hours Toward the End of the Week.

The best idea to accomplish this objective is to have both a stationary bicycle and a street bicycle. At the point when you can ride outside, when you can't, utilize the exercise bicycle in high apparatus (use a bicycle that gives the choice of attractive upper obstruction, which makes it difficult to pedal — as though you were going tough). Following ten minutes, you ought to sweat. If you ride in the city, go tough for in any event ten to fifteen minutes. Do this for around forty minutes each other day and for two hours toward the end of the week.

Bicycling might be healthier than running since it limits weight on the joints. In any case, a long-haul study indicated that long-separation running among healthy, more seasoned grown-ups were not related to osteoarthritis. So a physical issue brought about by long-separation running might be less regular than we would anticipate. Another investigation that followed 74,752 sprinters for a long time presumed that running diminished both weight and the danger of osteoarthritis.

Tailing one mainstay of life span (investigations of complex frameworks), we could infer that bicycling is desirable overrunning. Be that as it may, following another column (the study of disease transmission), running would have all the earmarks of being similarly acceptable. Its beneficial impacts, notwithstanding, may change after some time and may differ in people who are harmed, have joint harm, and keep on running. Along these lines, I would prescribe a bike as a first decision, yet running is additionally excellent if the breaking points portrayed underneath are followed.

Swimming is another great type of exercise, even though its valuable consequences for life span have gotten less investigation than those of running.

Utilize your Muscles.

Humans advanced as an animal type that strolls, runs, climbs trees and slopes, and uses an assortment of muscles regularly. Presently individuals use lifts and elevators rather than stairs, drive rather than walk, use dishwashers and clothes washers as opposed to washing dishes and garments by hand, purchase food as opposed to developing it, and contract individuals to do even minor fix work around the house as opposed to fixing things ourselves.

Each muscle of the body should be often utilized because muscles develop and keep up or gain quality just because of being tested. Climbing rapidly six flights of stairs can cause leg torment, mainly If you haven't done it in quite a while. That agony is proof of minor injury to your muscles. Within sight of adequate measures of proteins, muscle injury prompts the initiation of "muscle satellite cells" and, in the end, to muscle development. Muscles can be marginally harmed and revamped by doing basic regular errands that are testing. A minor injury can transform into a significant injury if the weight in weight-bearing exercise is excessively high or If you effectively keep re-harming excited muscle or ligament. Muscle preparation must be adjusted to dodge both acute wounds and the moderate, constant harm that accompanies disregarding agony and proceeding to put weight on a harmed joint.

Five of the Best Exercises You Can Ever Do

If you're not a contender or veritable exerciser — and you

need to work out so that your health or to fit in your pieces of clothing better — the rec focus scene can be alarming and overpowering. What are the best exercises for me? By what means will I find the time?

Anyway, most likely, the best physical exercises for your body don't require the rec focus or solicitation that you get adequately fit to run a long separation race. These "exercises" can do for your health. They'll help screen your weight, improve your equality and extent of development, strengthen your bones, secure your joints, thwart bladder control issues, and even stay away from memory mishaps.

Despite your age or health level, these exercises are the most flawlessly awesome exercises you can do and will help you with getting alive and well and lower your risk for ailment:

1. Swimming

You may call swimming the perfect exercise. "Swimming is useful for individuals with joint irritation since it's less weight-bearing. The water daintiness supports your body and removes the strain anguishing joints so you can move them even more efficiently.

It was found that swimming can improve your mental state and sets you feeling much improved. Water heart invigorating exercise is another decision. These classes help you with expanding calories and tone.

2. Judo

This Chinese military craftsmanship that combines

advancement and loosening up is helpful for both body and mind. It's been assigned, "thought to move." Tai chi contains the movement of easy advancements, and one changing effectively into the accompanying. The classes are offered at various levels; yoga is accessible — and significant — for people, everything being equivalent and health levels. It is exceptionally helpful for progressively settled people since balance is a massive piece of health, and equality is something we lose as we get increasingly prepared.

Take a class to help you with starting and become acquainted with the ideal structure.

3. Quality Planning

On the off chance that you acknowledge that quality getting ready is a macho, solid development, reevaluate. Lifting light loads won't hamburger up your muscles, yet it will keep them strong. If you don't use muscles, they will lose their quality after some time.

The muscle, in like manner, devours calories. The more muscle you have, the more calories you devour, so it's easier to keep up your weight. As another exercise, quality planning may moreover help shield with a braining limit in later years.

Before starting a weight planning program, make sure to get comfortable with the ideal structure. Start light, with just a few pounds. You should have the choice to lift the heaps on numerous occasions, no problem at all. Following a large portion of a month, increase that by a pound or two. On the off chance that you can, without quite a bit of a stretch, lift the heaps through the entire extent of development in an overabundance of various occasions, move to some degree heavier weight.

4. Walking

Walking is essential yet powerful. It can help you with staying trim, improve cholesterol levels, strengthen bones, hold beat under tight limitations, lift your perspective, and lower your peril for different ailments (diabetes and coronary disease, for example). Various examinations have shown that walking and other physical exercises can even improve memory and contradict age-related memory disasters.

All you need is a well-fitting and reliable pair of shoes. Start with walking around ten to15 minutes in a steady progression. After some time, you can start to walk progressively remote and speedier until you're walking about 30 to an hour on most days of the week.

5. Kegel Exercises

These exercises won't help you with looking better, yet they achieve something likewise as critical — sustain the pelvic floor muscles that support the bladder. Strong pelvic floor muscles can go far toward thwarting incontinence. While various women think about Kegels, these exercises can benefit men too.

To do a Kegel exercise adequately, press the muscles you would use to shield yourself from passing pee or gas. Hold the withdrawal for a couple of moments, by then release. Make a point to extricate up your pelvic floor muscles after the narrowing thoroughly. Repeat on different occasions. Endeavor to do four to five sets every day.

An enormous number of the things we achieve for amusement (and work) think about exercise. Raking the yard thinks about physical activity. So do traditional moving and playing with your youngsters or grandkids. For whatever time frame that you're doing some sort of oxygen expending exercise for on any occasion 30 minutes of the day, and you fuse two days of solidarity getting ready seven days, you can see yourself as a "working" person.

CHAPTER NINE

RESILIENCE AND WABI-SABI

Life is erratic. Furthermore, that is alright. Grasp it. When nothing is sure, the sky is the limit! Your arrangements for tomorrow, one month from now or one year from now, may not unfurl as you anticipate. It's imperative to make arrangements and proceed onward. Landon Donovan once stated, "Life isn't great, obviously. However, we as a whole know it's how you respond to things that matter."

A flaw is the fundamental standard of *Wabi-Sabi*, the Japanese way of thinking of tolerating your blemishes and capitalizing on life.

"*Wabi*" is said to be characterized as "provincial effortlessness" or "downplayed class," with attention on atoning it down would be the ideal mindset.

"*Sabi*" is meant "enjoying the flawed."

The concept of wabi-sabi is vast and practically challenging to distill in a single post, yet can, without much of a stretch, be applied just to moments of regular day-to-day existence. The constant quest for flawlessness — in assets, connections, accomplishments — frequently prompts pressure, uneasiness, melancholy, and rushed judgment. This is the place wabi-sabi welcomes an interruption. The Japanese way of thinking urges us to concentrate on the gifts covering up in our everyday lives and praising the status quo as opposed to how they ought to be. Wabi-sabi prizes credibility.

Wabi-Sabi is a lifestyle that acknowledges and acknowledges multifaceted nature while simultaneously values straightforwardness.

In Zen theory, there are seven tasteful standards in accomplishing wabi-sabi:

- *Kanso* — effortlessness
- *Fukinsei* — asymmetry or inconsistency
- *Shibumi* — excellence in the downplayed
- *Shizen* — instinctive nature without affectation
- *Yugen* — unpretentious beauty
- *Datsuzoku* — freeness
- *Seijaku* — peacefulness

The ageless astuteness of wabi-sabi is more pertinent now than at any time in recent memory for present-day life, as we look for significance and satisfaction past realism. Wabi-sabi resembles moderation with a conscious decision. The concept has its underlying foundations in the traditional Japanese tea function. A typical clarification is the case of an all-around adored teacup made by a craftsman's hands, broke or chipped by regular use. Such follows the onlooker that nothing is lasting — even fixed articles are liable to change.

An incredible case of wabi-sabi in imagination is the craft of kintsugi, where split earthenware is loaded up with gold tidied finish as an approach to grandstand the excellence of its age and harm as opposed to concealing it. The flaw isn't covered up yet featured. This isn't to state the Craftsman was messy (wabi-sabi isn't a reason for poor craftsmanship). Wabi-sabi causes one to notice the breaks in a teacup as a significant aspect of the magnificence of the article. It is contended that flaws are important for full energy about the item and the world. We, in our human flaws, are repulsed by the idea since everything is evident from the beginning, and there is no recommendation of the unbounded.

Wabi-sabi is all over; you simply need to realize what to look like and what to do to grasp the concept in your life. The splits in the old teacup are viewed as resources instead of defects. Wabi-sabi is an alternate sort of looking, another kind of mindset. It's the genuine acknowledgment of discovering excellence in things as they may be.

What Does It Take to Grasp Wabi-Sabi in Your Life?

You don't get cash or unique abilities to value your flaws and benefit as much as possible from life. Bringing wabi-sabi into your life doesn't require some money, preparation, or uncommon aptitudes. It takes a brain sufficiently calm to acknowledge quieted excellence, courage not to fear exposed state, readiness to recognize things as they are — without ornamentation. It relies upon the capacity to back off, to move the equalization from doing to being, to acknowledging instead of consummating.

Wabi-sabi is tied in with tolerating yourself and expanding on what you as of now have in life. Holding onto wabi-sabi is as simple (or as troublesome) as understanding and tolerating yourself — flaws whatnot. It's tied in with being empathetic with yourself as you may be and expanding on whatever that is — not hotly attempting to modify yourself to act like something different altogether.

Today, energy about the things we have, individuals we love, and the encounters we have the chance to mesh into our lives is losing esteem. Wabi-sabi speaks to a valuable reserve of knowledge that qualities serenity, harmony, magnificence, and blemish and can reinforce your resilience even with realism. It tenderly movements you to unwind, slow down, advance back from the riotous present-day world and discover enjoyment and gratitude in all that you do. Set forth plainly, wabi-sabi authorizes you to act naturally. Grasp the flawlessness of being incompletely you.

From the previous, it is evident that the "Wabi" reasonableness—the structure and soul of wabi-sabi—generally started as a tasteful convenience to the real disastrous factors of the day. There are equals presently. Progressively, we can make out the dim diagrams of calamitous situations to come. It is anticipated that more and greater atmosphere-related occasions will meet calamitously with a growing worldwide populace. How far will our material assets stretch? After the harm is over and over gathered up, will the greater part of us be constrained into smaller and smaller living conditions, with less and progressively unobtrusive items?

This need not be unfortunate. The magnificence of wabi-sabi is established in unobtrusiveness—even poverty—that is richly seen. The tasteful delights of wabi-sabi rely upon demeanor and practice to such an extent or more than on the materiality itself. Nuance and subtlety are at wabi-sabi's heart. Wabi-sabi lives in the subtle and neglected subtleties, in the minor and the covered up, in the conditional and vaporous. Certain brain habits are required to value these characteristics: tranquility, mindfulness, and astuteness. If these are absent, wabi-sabi is undetectable.

Wabi-sabi is a Japanese concept, the magnificence that is temporary, flawed, and fragmented. Wabi-sabi has an association with a training known as *kintsugi,* or *kintsukuroi,* the specialty of fixing broken ceramics with polish blended in with gold, silver, or platinum. The thought is that the breaks are presently a piece of the defective work, not something to be concealed away or secured.

CHAPTER TEN

HOW TO FIND OUR IKIGAI

Justifiably, when individuals become acquainted with the concept of ikigai, they need to take a plunge, handle characterizing it as a discrete undertaking. At that point, jump energetically dependent on the aftereffects of that venture. In any case, comprehend that making sense of your ikigai doesn't occur incidentally. Instead of being something that you mystically find, your purpose unfurls and will develop after some time.

That is not a reason to kick back and expect your ikigai to introduce itself. Discovering it requires an eagerness for profound self-investigation and experimentation, and there are approaches to deal with that. Astute reflection, joined with move make, can assist you with uncovering how your qualities, qualities, and abilities can be brought to the closer view to help you with discovering all the more important in your life and vocation—and the equalization of ikigai.

Here's a 5-advance procedure on the most proficient method to encourage the correct attitude to let your ikigai create.

1. Start with questions.

Snatch a diary and ask yourself the accompanying inquiries:

- What do you love? (These address your energy.)
- What would you say you are acceptable at? (These address your calling.)
- What does the world need? (These address your central goal.)

- What would you be able to get paid for? (These address your livelihood.)

You don't need to drive yourself to concoct replies at a time. It's increasingly beneficial to require some investment.

Through the span of a couple of days or weeks, accept notes as thoughts and bits of knowledge come to you. In particular, be drastically fair with yourself. Try not to be reluctant to write down whatever rings a bell, regardless of how insane or silly it may appear to be at present.

If those inquiries aren't starting as a lot of understanding as you might want, attempt these:

- What might you want to see change on the planet?
- What, in your life as it is currently, fulfills you?
- Why do you get up in the first part of the day?
- Have you had any life-changing moments that given a lightning electrical jolt?

Make sure to incorporate other life or professional encounters that altogether illuminate your qualities.

After you've addressed these inquiries keenly, begin to search for designs. What sorts of topics are obvious? Are there clear crossing points among classes, or do they appear to be different? If unmistakable connections aren't apparent, don't stress — that is ordinary. This procedure will require some serious energy.

It tends to be difficult to see yourself impartially, which is the place getting outside input comes in. I asked loved ones to namelessly mention to me what they saw as my three best characteristics. Taking evaluations like Strengths Finder and the VIA character qualities overview likewise helped me recognize (and make a jargon around) my abilities and characteristics.

Unexpectedly, characteristics about myself that I underestimated were exactly what others saw as exceptional and significant. Rather than minimizing my skill for sympathy, their remarks bumped me to look further at how I could use my affectability as a quality and turn my profession to concentrate on training, educating, and composing.

2. Guide it Out.

Mapping out your responses to the inquiries above is useful, particularly If you feel stuck. There is a wide range of approaches to make a guide; explore different avenues regarding whatever sounds good to you.

It can be helpful to draw interlocking circles for every classification (a Venn diagram, similar to the one above). In contrast, others like to outline on a quadrant, composing thoughts that meet numerous criteria close to the crossing point of the tomahawks. The guide doesn't need to be lovely. It simply needs to sort out your musings. This is a living report, so it will change and advance after some time. As you begin to test your ikigai in reality, you will strike out things and include others.

Since I'm considerably more of an experiential student as opposed to a legitimate organizer, I invested some energy thoroughly considering and mapping out my Ideal Day. This includes portraying what your optimal average workday resembles in however much detail as could reasonably be expected (recollect, an ikigai is even-minded). As such, you imagine what an exciting day living your ikigai may involve.

At the point when I experienced this exercise, it was enlightening. I understood I'd love just to begin my day at the rec center, trailed by telecommuting. I'd shift back and forth between long periods of profound work on creative ventures and days loaded up with training customers. After some time, these gradual changes include—and draw you nearer to living an all the more by and by meaningful life.

3. Check Whether it Feels Right.

Regardless of whether you're holding a rundown or a guide or something different from the means above, reflect and do a proper check.

These are advantageous inquiries to pose, regardless of whether you decided your ikigai forty years back or you're simply finding out about the concept now. In case you're on an underlying ikigai certainty discovering venture, coordinating intuitive pushes with rationale-driven reasoning can prompt a more profound, increasingly cognizant feeling of purpose.

Start by posting three unique portrayals of your conceivable ikigai. The first ought to mirror your present way, while the second and third ought to reflect what you'd pick if cash or others' desires didn't make a difference. The vast majority of my customers want to utilize the worksheet accessible on the Designing Your Life site, or you can portray your own. At that point, rank how you feel about each cigar way dependent on:

- How much you like it

- How certain you with it
- Does it fits with your life and work

4. Test It

The result of finding your ikigai is in living it out. Like any goal, it doesn't occur through contemplation alone. You need to focus on predictable activity to gain ground—and to cause modifications en route to keep on to develop. When you've shown up at a working thought regarding your ikigai, it's an excellent opportunity to make some move, in reality, to test if following this life purpose is something you will discover essential and satisfying.

This may include moving needs or investigating new bearings. For instance, possibly you select to travel less and organize family time. Maybe you start another business that joins various interests. You may wind up changing vocations totally if your present center doesn't cover with your ikigai.

At the point when you start to make strides towards your objective, your ikigai will be tried, and that is a generally beautiful thing. Creator Neil Pasricha recommends running your ikigai through the Saturday Morning Test: Make sure your ikigai is something you'd end up happily attracted to on a beautiful day away from work.

5. Fabricate Your Emotionally Supportive Network

Likewise, with the vast majority of life's changes, it's essential to have support while deliberately building up your feeling of ikigai. If you've chosen to move in the direction of another vocation — transforming a side undertaking into a full-time attempt, for example—it's critical to have tutors managing you, just as to have caring individuals in your corner.

Develop a relationship with somebody who has made a relative professional change. Get some information about their experience making the jump and which parts of it were the most testing and the most fulfilling?

Updates are making progress toward finding your "sweet spot."

Attempt to be Non-Critical About Your Ikigai.

If you discover your feeling of purpose through a commitment to your profession, that is magnificent. It doesn't imply that your family, companions, or otherworldliness are not imperative to you and that you shouldn't set aside a few minutes for them. It necessarily means that an enormous piece of "what you live for" originates from the feeling of remuneration and achievement you get from the things you take on through your employment and calling.

Few Out of Every Odd Moment of Consistently Will Be Joyful.

Remember that even as you seek after your feeling of purpose, a few out of every odd moment of consistently will be simple or even enjoyable. Notwithstanding the progressions you've made in your profession or life, you'll likely despise everything you need to make tradeoffs and bargains now and again. In case you're associated with your feeling of purpose more often than not, though, you'll be more robust and keep awful days in context.

Let Your Ikigai Be Your Guide.

An ikigai, here and there, resembles a compass. Adjusting your activities to "what you live for" causes you to explore high life points and low points. As your vocation develops and you're given more chances, you can depend on your ikigai to guide you the correct way.

Make sure to assess your feeling of happiness and purpose at each progression en route. By looking for development that accommodates your sense of purpose, you seek health and happiness too.

CONCLUSION

Discovering the key to Japanese individuals' record-breaking long life and excellent health is no easy task. Still, if armed with sound sources and perseverance to better oneself, one can practice said lifestyle with ease. The ethos of ikigai is overwhelming the West. This ethos, the "purposes behind being," has been drilled in Japan for many years. It's such a lifestyle that it's underestimated. In the Japanese language, ikigai is utilized in different settings and can apply to small ordinary things just as to huge objectives and accomplishments. It is such a common word that individuals use it in day-by-day life calmly, without monitoring its having any exceptional criticalness. Above all, ikigai is conceivable without your fundamentally being active in your expert life. Right now, it is an extremely law-based concept, saturated with a festival of the assorted variety of life. The facts demonstrate that having ikigai can bring about progress. However, achievement is anything but an essential condition for having ikigai. It is available to all of us.

Ikigai lives in the domain of small things. The morning air, some espresso, the beam of daylight, and the kneading of octopus meat. Just the individuals who can perceive the wealth of this entire range honestly acknowledge and enjoy it. This is an essential exercise of ikigai. In reality, as we know it, where our incentive as individuals and our feeling of self-esteem is resolved principally by our prosperity, numerous individuals are feeling the squeeze. You may think that any worth framework you have is just commendable and defended If it converts into substantial accomplishments – an advancement, for instance, or a rewarding venture.

All things considered, unwind! You can have ikigai, an

incentive to live by, without fundamentally substantiating yourself in that way. Saying this doesn't imply that it will come to no problem at all. Moreover, the death rate for individuals who addressed 'yes' to the ikigai question was substantially lower than for the individuals who sent 'no.' The lower price was the aftereffect of their being at a lower danger of cardiovascular infection. Curiously, there was no critical change in the threat of malignant growth for individuals who addressed 'yes' contrasted with the individuals who sent 'no' to the ikigai question.

For what reason did the individuals with ikigai likewise have a diminished danger of experiencing cardiovascular illness? The upkeep of good health includes many elements. It is hard to state unquestionably what variables are at last mindful however the decrease of cardiovascular ailment would propose that the individuals who have ikigai are bound to exercise since commitment to physical exercises are known to diminish the danger of cardiovascular disease. To be sure, the Ōsaki study found that the individuals who addressed positively about ikigai exercised more than the individuals who gave an adverse reaction. Ikigai gives your life a purpose while giving you the coarseness to continue.

Finding Your Ikigai

Your purpose and explanation behind being will be one of a kind and uncommon to you. For a few, their Ikigai is self-evident. It's enthusiasm or work that they grasp and devote themselves entirely to consistently. Others may be looking for their purpose, despite everything attempting to figure out what it is they esteem. In case you're despite everything looking, here are specific ways you can try to decide your purpose in life.

Keep a journal – journaling when and why you felt you've felt satisfaction or achievement can help recognize what's critical to you.

Consider what you're appreciative of – before you rest, express so anyone might hear five things that caused you to feel thankful that day. Search for ongoing ideas between these occasions.

Surrender things – take a week or more extended without specific things in your life. Start with those you think maybe an exercise in futility, similar to TV or online experience. What you usually incline toward when you aren't given speedy amusement fixes is most likely uncommon to you.

Converse with the individuals who realize you best – your loved ones may know you superior to anything you know yourself. Ask their sentiment on what they figure your Ikigai could be. You'd be amazed at what they may state.

PRACTICAL GUIDE TO KAIZEN

HOW TO ACHIEVE YOUR GOALS AND INCREASE YOUR PRODUCTIVITY THROUGH MINI HABITS, THE JAPANESE WAY

BY

MARK MORIMOTO

INTRODUCTION

Kaizen, which is about continuous improvement, has been known to have existed after the Second World War. Today, it is utilized to improve different sorts of processes associated with designing, manufacturing, the board, and other supporting operations in the business. This is additionally applied in social insurance places, life guiding, banking, government, and even psychotherapy. Presently, if you will utilize this in your business, yet you are very hesitant to begin due to the reactions you may have found out about it, think about this as activities that you can perform to improve their capacities ceaselessly. Everybody should take an interest here, beginning from the CEOs up to the slightest degree of representatives. Kaizen has an incredible breadth as it presently applies to processes that cross the association's restrictions into the store network itself. These may incorporate coordination and buying activities. With the end goal for you to comprehend this well, you may require a case of kaizen execution.

To execute the kaizen approach, what you need is a closed group that has been predictable with the lean systems' utilization. Regularly, the individuals right now need to experience some training to begin encouraging the kaizen methodology into your association. Kaizen is an activity that you need to perform day by day, and what you ought to do here is to give a reason which ought to go past improvement. When actualized effectively, Kaizen will empower you to acculturate the workplace just as eliminate all the processes that need a ton of work from your representatives, which can be about mental and physical activities. Kaizen will likewise show your kin how they can perform errands in a fast manner through examinations. They have to apply here is a logical method that will help them figure out how to eliminate waste in the processes.

Right now, kaizen usage, you should know the cycle of kaizen. This will initially begin with the process of standardizing an activity. At that point, you should quantify that specific activity. This implies you should give the cycle time just as the measure of the in-process stock. At that point, you should ascertain the estimations against goals or necessities that you said for motivation for improvement. The fourth step is to make a few thoughts to ensure that you will have the option to meet the needs and increment profitability. This will, at that point, lead you into the as good as every task in your business.

When you actualize kaizen approach, you ought to be that there ought to be advisors in the offices so the groups of representatives will have the option to execute their assignment well, especially with the use of kaizen. Ensure that there is a chosen process that is in the center when you manage kaizen. The specialists should give a report that will provide insights concerning the assistance of the association's actual kaizen occasion. You can have the same number of groups as you need, which cover different objective processes in your business will; however, be sure that the kaizen plans have been educated to the territory workforce accountable for the groups.

CHAPTER ONE

INTRODUCING KAIZEN

Kaizen is a powerful way of thinking that can be applied to pretty much every aspect of life. The Japanese word Kaizen interprets straightforwardly into "improvement," while in idea, it means continuous development, advancement, and improvement. It is a process of continuously evaluating new things to continue improving one's job or lifestyle. Kaizen in the workplace engages representatives to screen their work and to bring up territories of improvement that, like this, would require small advances that would, therefore, create specific outcomes. These substantial outcomes delivering small increases will slowly bring about significant strides for actual improvement when assembled.

The way of thinking likewise improves teamwork, as representatives additionally figure out how to pay particular minds to one another and to, in the end, counsel and create through the small units. The vast number of small advances made from these units, more Muda or waste, the adversary of profitability, would be eliminated. Kaizen was first successfully executed and utilized in the Toyota manufacturing plant in Japan, yet it's currently accessible to all ventures using an extensive Kaizen introduction. The kaizen introduction is a definitive material for training your representatives to work the Kaizen way.

The usual Kaizen introduction starts with the definition, characteristics, and principles of the way of thinking. It would viably present Kaizen as a way of thinking and afterward create Kaizen mindfulness in your workers through a complete conversation of its advantages and different sorts of its methodologies. Moreover, the average

Kaizen introduction means to grow enough mindfulness that they would have the option to comprehend what is required for a Kaizen occasion. What's more, when they can understand these prerequisites, they are educated to accumulate the tools (which are, for the most part, information). At the point when this is all together, they would then be able to take a stab at planning, supporting, and making an interest in an actual Kaizen venture.

A Kaizen introduction additionally ordinarily incorporates stable instances of Kaizen ventures from which the workers can also gain from and maybe base a portion of their plans. These models are more given to offer an opportunity for conversation on the processes and consequences of dynamic among coaches and learners.

What is Kaizen?

Various individuals, that are new to Lean Manufacturing will sooner or later wind up saying, "Kaizen? What is Kaizen? Am I not catching your meaning by Kaizen? What does Kaizen do?" Several terms and definitions ring a bell when discussing Kaizen. Kaizen is a Japanese expression signifying "Change to improve things" or "improvement." It is most usually converted into English as "Continuous Improvement." Kaizen is one of the messengers in Lean reasoning and requires control and constant re-assessment. It works on the premise that nothing can ever get great. There is continually something that can be improved.

Numerous methodologies originate from a specific piece of the world, and out of nowhere, they are adopted by multiple nations currently, including the United States. Concerning business, this is practically similar to a convention since it is significant for the business proprietors to discover and explore the freshest tactic on how they would have the option to help their organization and help make it one of the most regarded firms the planet. Japan has been known everywhere throughout the earth for its rich culture and customs. There are additionally conventional business practices in Japan, and one of the most well-known is kaizen. If this is the first occasion you have heard this term, you may ponder and ask, "What is kaizen?" Many people don't know that kaizen is being utilized in Japan and in different spots that are amazing as far as their impact in the business world, for example, the United States. So what is kaizen truly?

The primary kaizen definition is a Japanese custom that is adjusted by the Japanese culture to best suit the business condition they are by and by. Indeed, this is a Japanese expression, which means "getting great through change." Therefore, we can infer that kaizen is a method that comprises rebuilding and dealing with every single business aspect to guarantee the organization that it is consistently at its pinnacle productivity. In this way, to comprehend the response to the inquiry "what is kaizen" much more, we can discuss the five essential components wherein this is fundamentally established upon.

First is about the quality circles, which imply that there are bunches that would generally meet within the firm so the individuals would all be able to talk about the quality levels. These are worried about all the aspects of the tasks of the organization. The following component is improved confidence, which accepts that there should be solid resolve in the workforce. This is viewed as an important advance towards achieving long haul viability and proficiency, just as profitability. Kaizen is a Japanese methodology set as a critical activity to keep in touch with the representatives' spirit.

The third is about teamwork, which indicates that a trustworthy organization ought to have the option to arrange the representatives with the goal that each undertaking will be fruitful. The fundamental point here is to utilize kaizen to ensure that the organization will have the option to get the assistance that it requires for the workers and the supervisory crew as they take a gander at themselves and their activities in general. They will comprehend that they should work as a group, not as contenders. Fourth is close to home order wherein the group can't succeed except if they work with each other. Furthermore, every individual from the group should know their capacities and sharpen them without anyone else. There ought to likewise be responsibility by every representative for individual control. Ultimately, there ought to be recommendations for improvement. Every part ought to give their input, and the administration should affirm that problems are considered and tended to.

Kaizen on an organization scale can mean a few things. As a significant aspect of a continuous improvement culture, most organizations hold what is called Kaizen Events. These are commonly an activity that expels individuals from their daily assignments and spot them in a group to achieve an objective within three to five days. These are exceptionally focused on ventures with feasible outcomes, for example, moving machines so they can work more like each other for continuous flow, or planning and executing another lining system for a particular reason, or a SMED occasion, and so on. Regardless of the objective, the process is generally the equivalent: Plan, Do, Check, Act.

Plan, Do Check, Act (PDCA) was created by W. Edwards Deming and presented in Japan during the 1950s. It depends on the Scientific Method and is a forerunner to Six Sigma's DMAIC process (Define, Measure, Analyze, Improve, and Control). This is how PDCA separates:

- Plan - Develop a sound, very much idea out the objective (that can be accomplished with moderate exertion), and how to accomplish it.

- Do - Implement the thoughts and, additionally, changes expected to accomplish the objective, including training.
- Check - Review what you've done; be basic.
- Act – This depends on how the Check step went, continue these outcomes, or play out the entire PDCA cycle over once more.

You can see this is an unadulterated continuous improvement as the cycle can be finished again and again. The Toyota Production System has somewhat changed this language to be Plan, Try, Reflect, and Standardize. Different repetition, yet the same desires for process and results. Regularly, most Lean training and assets characterize Kaizen's two sorts: System or Flow Kaizen and Process Kaizen.

A System or Flow Kaizen manages a whole worth stream being assessed for chances of improvements and will ordinarily incorporate action from a few board degrees. A Process Kaizen is a concentrated improvement of a solitary process (or gatherings of a similar operation). This kind of Kaizen will typically incorporate a cross-functional group committed to improving that individual process.

Both of these sorts of Kaizen are plentiful in any valuable Lean undertaking and are at the very heart of those associations. Working within an organization that requires help to execute Lean can start to wear on your mind, mainly If you are the change specialist. For my whole expert vocation, I've needed to take on this job. You push and push each day for changes since you can see the waste sitting all around the plant and office, in piles of wasted stock and DMR'd materials to unimportant strides in itcm improvement processes. It's hard to keep an uplifting disposition.

After some time, I've figured out how to consolidate Kaizen's possibility into everything that I do. I make it a habit to express this word to myself repeatedly on various occasions during the day. While at work, it keeps me and opens my mind to believe that everything can be improved if we simply put forth a concentrated effort somewhat more. Presently, I will, in general, Implement Then Perfect, which is a decent, counterbalance definition (kind of) of Kaizen, while right off the bat in my vocation, I would invest an excessive amount of energy considering conceivable outcomes rather than merely doing. This makes better results and makes you think on a Results-Driven premise, which is how you need to remember - you will continually develop and improve - only like an organization that keeps up a stable Kaizen attitude.

On an individual level, use Kaizen to improve your life, and it will work its way into your expert vocation. Add it into your daily life with work out, dietary patterns, indecencies, and so forth. If you need to begin working out, start small and work from that point - include somewhat consistently. Those are small, steady improvements that work. If you overeat, attempt to eat one more minor nibble at one feast each other day, and in the long run, climb to 1 chomp for each dinner consistently. If you smoke and need to stop, cut back gradually, and your body will react well. These methods work for you, and similar kinds of stepwise improvements drive positive changes in your organization.

If you know somebody who professes to be great - they're most certainly not; indeed, even a great deal of the best individuals will reveal to you that they are not high and that that conviction is the thing that got them to where they are today - and it keeps them there. You might be thinking: "Won't that reasoning simply make me discouraged?" actually, no, it won't. When you permit yourself to see the imperfections that keep you down, you will be significantly more liable to conquer them. A decent proverb that I attempt to live by is: Always be cheerful, however never be fulfilled. That is the substance of Kaizen. It will carry continuous improvement to your life. That is Kaizen.

Kaizen - Continuous Improvement Process

It is said that at one Toyota factory, there are a million recommendations received from representatives consistently. So the inquiry is: How the administration of the Company can deal with such huge numbers of recommendations? The appropriate response is necessary: they do not deal with these proposals. Instead, they composed all representatives in a gathering of roughly five individuals. If one individual from the audience thinks, that individual presents it to different individuals from a group. If the Idea is adopted, they mostly go with it, without the requirement for additional endorsement. The particular case could be the circumstance when the Idea requires an enormous venture. This process of continuous improvement is called Kaizen.

This is a case of a base-up system of the continuous improvement process. This is how that is creating a gigantic pool of thoughts that can improve the association's viability and effectiveness. Kaizen supports the idea of worker strengthening. Kaizen is the administration approach that perceives workers' capability and does not require administrative endorsements for improvement activities. This is the system that significantly relies upon the social arrangement of an association. If the administration of an association accepts that workers are apathetic and bumbling, so there is a requirement for a stable controlling system, at that point, the Kaizen is beyond the realm of imagination.

The idea of Kaizen is process change and improvement through the vast number of small advances. This process is, at last, prompting an upper hand of an association. This implies an association will be increasingly gainful at the lower cost. At the same time, supervisors' primary job won't be to discover small improvements, however, to be centered around more significant changes.

The principle is the equivalent for the entire organization; however, it generally alludes to the organization's shop level. The attention is given to improving things as opposed to improving things. Kaizen requires a devoted, engaged, and multiskilling workforce that works with least of course an endorsement system. The Kaizen requires a propelled phase of networking. Groups should be framed rapidly, and they have to begin with their work in a brief timeframe. Networks of individuals who share regular encounters and problems should be supported. For the most part, these gatherings are making other thoughts and activities. Additionally, they defeat the obstructions innovatively.

By and large, the sharing of thoughts and Best Practice arrangements is significant. Tragically sharing of ideas isn't generally the situation. It is essential to discover the best approach to coordinate people's vitality and innovativeness into the network of individuals who manage the same problems. Within each association, there are a few limitations that oppose to Kaizen-like improvement process. The most widely recognized is Silo-figuring, which might be entombed departmentally or bury organization, for associations that work in more nations. The regular obstruction is worry about extra costs that may show up. An improvement now and again requires ventures expected to direct the change to improve the association's proficiency. At long last, there is obstruction of individual directors to lose control over the processes.

Kaizen isn't something that is anything but difficult to execute. First, it must begin from the top and step by step to move the rationale of the entire idea to the least level—the

Kaizen is a continuous improvement process that should be energized. Today, every association is confronted with the quickly evolving condition, market, and purchaser's inclination. Just the association that is proficient at changing rapidly can remain serious. The Kaizen is conclusively the idea that can bolster this change capacity; like this, it ought to be presented and upheld.

The Similarities between Balanced Scorccards and Kaizen

Numerous business people have been intrigued by both the BSC and kaizen. These two business systems of approach are unquestionably the absolute most confided in plans today. A few business pioneers are known to have actualized these two on their organization system. Even if they have various extensions and centers, the balanced scorecard and kaizen share a couple of things in like manner. There are undoubtedly a few likenesses between adjusted scorecards and Kaizen that the clients should think about. The first is that they are amazingly adaptable, implying that they can be utilized in any office or division in the organization. You can place this in the money-related office, the deals, or even the manufacturing division. Additionally, connected here is a hierarchical framework that can be applied to the two structures. There is the thing that we call the corporate scorecard, and there is a hierarchical strategy for kaizen.

BSC and kaizen additionally focus on specific things. In the balanced scorecard, four perspectives are being considered: the clients, the financials, the learning and development, and the inner processes. The last is the primary worry of kaizen. You may have caught wind of the *Gemba* kaizen, which relates to the kaizen applied in the workplace itself. The *gembutsu* is gotten from the Japanese word, which implies the unmistakable items that are found in the Gemba. These can incorporate the machines, the tools, the rejects, and others.

Another from the likenesses between adjusted scorecards and Kaizen is that these two can be considered as estimating tools for businesses. The balanced scorecard gives the organization's exact yet short presentation on the referenced four points of view. Then again, kaizen is about estimating the improvement of the business processes when contrasted with its typical tactics. The disposal of wasteful processes is one of the leading destinations here.

Presently, regardless of whether you have just gotten the outcomes originating from the BSC and the continuous improvement system, you will understand that there is a requirement for you to refresh them both continually. This is another of the similitudes between adjusted scorecards and Kaizen. You are required to gauge and get the basic snippets of data originating from these two with the goal that you can effectively screen the viability of your business. Thus, the BSC and kaizen are not just for your organization's present circumstance, yet they are both for vital actions, which imply that they are made for the eventual fate of the business.

Both the reasonable scorecard and the kaizen approach utilize key execution pointers that empower the supervisors to monitor their association's strength. The BSC's KPIs depend on the four points of view again, while in kaizen, you have quality, cost, exertion, profitability, and timetable or time. At last, the best in the likenesses between adjusted scorecards and Kaizen is that the organization can get profits from them. The points of interest that you can are various; however, they can be abridged into 3Rs, which relate to doing things the correct way, doing the right things, and performing them at the perfect time.

Five S of Kaizen

"Kaizen" alludes to a Japanese word that signifies "improvement" or "change to improve things." Kaizen is characterized as a continuous exertion by every representative (from the CEO to handle staff) to guarantee the improvement of everything equal and systems of a specific association. Work for a Japanese organization, and you would before long acknowledge how a lot of significance they provide for Kaizen's process. The Kaizen method encourages Japanese organizations to eclipse every other contender by holding fast to specific set arrangements and rules to eliminate absconds and guarantee long haul unrivaled quality and, in the end, consumer loyalty.

Kaizen works on the accompanying fundamental principle.

"Change is for acceptable."

Kaizen signifies "continuous improvement of processes and elements of an association through change." In a layman's language, Kaizen gets continuous small improvements in the general processes and inevitably points towards the association's prosperity. Japanese feel that numerous small permanent changes in the systems and arrangements bring successful outcomes than barely any significant changes.

Kaizen process focuses on continuous improvement of operations in the manufacturing area and every other office. Executing Kaizen tools isn't the obligation of a solitary individual; however, it includes each part that is legitimately connected with the association. Regardless of his/her assignment or level in order, each person needs to contribute by consolidating small improvements and changes in the system.

Following are the primary components of Six Sigma:

· Teamwork

· Personal Discipline

· Improved Morale

· Quality Circles

· Suggestions for Improvement

"Five S" of Kaizen is a systematic methodology that prompts idiot-proof systems, standard approaches, rules, and guidelines to offer ascent to a sound work culture at the association. You would scarcely locate an individual speaking to a Japanese organization miserable or disappointed. Japanese workers never talk sick about their association. Indeed, Kaizen's process assumes a significant job in representative satisfaction and consumer loyalty through small continuous changes and dispensing with surrenders. Kaizen tools offer ascent to an efficient workplace, which brings about better profitability and yields better outcomes. It additionally prompts workers who emphatically feel connected towards the association.

Let us comprehend the five S in Detail:

1. SEIRI - SEIRI represents Sort Out. As indicated by Seiri, workers should sift through and sort out things well. Mark the things as "Essential", "Basic", "Generally Important", "Not required now", "Futile, etc. Toss what everything is pointless. Keep aside what everything isn't required right now. Things that are basic and most significant ought to be kept at a sheltered spot.
2. SECTION - Section intends to arrange. Research says that workers waste a portion of their valuable time scanning for things and essential documents.

Each element ought to have its own space and should be kept at its place as it were.

3. SEO - "SEISO" signifies sparkle in the workplace. The workplace should be kept clean—De-mess your workstation. Essential documents ought to be held in legitimate envelopes and records. Use cupboards and drawers to store your things.

4. SEIKETSU-SEIKETSU alludes to Standardization. Each association needs to have specific standard rules and set strategies to guarantee prevalent quality for them.

5. SHITSUKE or Self Discipline - Workers need to regard the association's approaches and hold fast to rules and guidelines. Self-restraint is fundamental. Do not go to the office in casuals. Follow work methods, and do not neglect to convey your personality cards to work. It gives you a feeling of pride and regard for the association.

Kaizen centers on continuous small improvements and, in this way, gives prompt outcomes.

Origins and History of Kaizen

Kaizen History

Kaizen's history starts after World War II when Toyota first executed quality circles in quite a whole production process. This was affected to some degree by American business and quality administration educators who visited the nation. A quality circle is a gathering of workers playing out the equivalent or similar work, who meet routinely to recognize, dissect, and take care of work-related problems. This progressive idea became extremely famous in Japan during the 1950s and kept on existing as Kaizen bunches just as comparable worker investment plans. The term Kaizen got acclaimed the world over through the works of Masaaki Imai.

Masaaki Imai (conceived, 1930) is a Japanese hierarchical scholar and the board specialist, known for his work on quality administration, explicitly on Kaizen. In 1985, the Kaizen Institute Consulting Group (KICG) was established to enable western organizations to present Kaizen's ideas, systems, and tools. At present, the Kaizen Institute group has applied for the lean methodology and kaizen training courses across all intents and purposes, all business areas worldwide.

Masaaki Imai distributed two critical books on the business process the board "Kaizen: Japanese soul of improvement" (1985), which advanced the Kaizen idea in the West, and Gemba Kaizen: A Commonsense, Low-Cost Approach to Management (1997).

Kaizen Event

In present-day utilization, kaizen is intended to address a specific issue throughout seven days, alluded to as a "kaizen rush" or "kaizen occasion." A kaizen occasion is an engaged advancement venture that can achieve leap forward improvements in a short measure of time, around 2-10 days in scope. Kaizen occasions must have a clear, brief goal alongside promptly accessible assets and fast outcomes. This guarantees the results are critical, clear, and quick to advance the age of proceeded with eagerness and satisfaction.

Ten Principles of Kaizen

The Kaizen method follows ten explicit principles, which are depicted beneath:

1. Improve everything continuously.
2. Abolish old, customary ideas.
3. Accept no reasons and get things going.
4. Say no to the norm of executing new methods and accepting they will work.

5. If something isn't right, make it right.
6. Empower everybody to partake in problem settling.
7. Get data and sentiments from different individuals.
8. Before deciding, ask "why" multiple times to find a workable pace cause. (5 Why Method)
9. Be efficient - Set aside cash through small improvements and spend a good deal on further developments.
10. Recollect that improvement has no restrictions. Try always to improve.

Kaizen method endeavors toward flawlessness by killing waste *(Muda)* in the workplace *(Gemba)*.

The objective of kaizen is production without residues by improving standardized activities and processes. Modern designer Taiichi Ohno, the dad of the Toyota Production System, saw that there is an 80% misfortune in each process, and the estimation of the process is under 20%.

The Seven Wastes (Muda)

A segment of micro-processes working as a component of the full process does not change an item that the shopper is happy to pay for. In the wake of breaking down manufacturing processes, Taiichi Ohno had the option to distinguish which steps include worth and which ones do not. Subsequently, he built up a superior path for associations to recognize waste with his "Seven Wastes" model. These wastes include:

1. Delay, pausing, or time went through in line with no worth being included. An enormous piece of an individual item's life is spent holding on to be worked on.
2. Producing more than you need. Overproduction usually covers up or potentially creates all the others. It prompts abundance stock, which at that

point requires the use of assets on extra room and conservation. These activities do not profit the client.

3. Over-processing or undertaking non-esteem included activity. Over-processing happens when more work is performed on a piece than what is required by the client.
4. Transportation. Each time an item is moved, it stands the danger of being harmed, lost, postponed, and so forth as an expense for no additional worth.
5. Unnecessary development or movement. Movement alludes to the harm that the production process delivers on the element that makes the item. This might be either after some time (mileage for gear and tedious strain wounds for workers) or during discrete occasions (mishaps that harm hardware and additionally harm workers).
6. Inventory. Whether it is as crude materials, work-in-progress, or completed merchandise, it speaks to a capital cost that has not yet delivered a salary, either by the maker or for the customer.
7. Production of Defects. Imperfections cause additional expenses for reworking the part and can, in some cases, bring about doubling the loss of one single item.

Gemba Kaizen

Genba (additionally Romanized as Gemba) is a Japanese expression signifying "the genuine spot." In lean manufacturing, the possibility of Gemba is that the problems are apparent, and the best improvement thoughts will originate from heading off to the Gemba (the factory floor in manufacturing). The Gemba walk takes lean administration to the bleeding edges to search for waste and chances to practice Gemba kaizen or practical shop-floor improvement.

The term Gemba, in universal practice, turned out to be

generally known after productions about the Toyota quality administration system. In practice, if a problem happens, the designers must go to the source to comprehend the problem's full impact, gathering information from all sources. Japanese dynamic principle varies from a conventional American administration approach where choices are regularly made remotely.

The brilliant rule of Gemba the board, called the 5-Gemba principles, is as per the following:

1. When trouble (irregularity) emerges, go to Gemba first.
2. Check with *gembutsu* (machines, tools, rejects, and client grumblings).
3. Take impermanent countermeasures on the spot.
4. Find out the underlying driver. By rehashing the inquiry "why" a few times, you can discover the underlying driver of the problem.
5. Standardize for the avoidance of repeat.

In the present circumstance of dealing with numerous undertakings and settling on choices snappier, directors regularly attempt to apply the most recent significant expense advancements to deal with problems that can be explained with a practical, straightforward approach. The kaizen method includes the utilization of the right tools, checklists, and strategies. It doesn't require the venture of a lot of cash yet offers considerable advantages to any business. Simultaneously, If you are a fan of advancements and comprehend the kaizen approach is precisely what your association needs to actualize, you can adopt some online instrument supporting the methodology. Kanbanchi is one of such tools.

Who made Kaizen?

One individual or organization didn't make Kaizen, yet

instead, various specialists teamed up and made tools that would result in the long run advance to what we know as Kaizen. W. Edwards Deming, an American administration advisor, and analyst, based upon Walter A. Shewhart's ideas of measurable process control to create the board ideas with cycles and the possibility of improvement. Following World War II, Deming was sent to Japan to contemplate agrarian production problems and different issues in the country harmed by the war.

Deming and different specialists from America teamed up with Japanese business directors to think of better approaches to build profitability in the office and improve item quality for the customer. In 1951, the Deming Circle, which of four stages that cycle through the structure, production, deals, and research, was reworked by the Japanese and was formed into the Plan > Did> Check > Act (PDCA) Cycle. The PDCA cycle is a crucial segment of Kaizen.

Toyota's Impact

The Toyota Motor Corporation is a Japanese organization known for effectively tackling the lessons of Deming and others. Kaizen's primary trace was when Toyota utilized quality circles during the 1950s as a significant aspect of the manufacturing process. Quality control circles are gatherings of representatives with the equivalent or similar job who get together all the time to characterize, investigate, and discover answers for issues identified with their work. In the long run, the utilization of value circles. Deming's lessons and the Training Within Industry (TWI) program all prompted the Toyota Production System's advancement.

Masaaki Imai, a Japanese hierarchical scholar, and the board expert, examined the Toyota Production System and its Lean principles and was the first to acquaint the possibility of

Kaizen with both Europe and North America. Imai went on to establish the Kaizen Institute in 1985 to advance Kaizen around the world.

Kaizen is presently utilized worldwide by an assortment of organizations. The possibility of continuous improvement supports workers from all levels to include problem understanding and expands an association's profitability significantly. While this is only a brief and dense form of Kaizen's history, it is essential to realize the critical characters associated with Kaizen's origination: Deming, Toyota, and Imai.

History of Kaizen - The Key Players

Walter A. Shewhart

Walter A. Shewhart was an American analyst, physicist, and Engineer. During the 1920s, while he worked at Bell Laboratories, Shewhart made the ideas of the measurable control of processes, and Shewhart additionally built up the control outline device.

Measurable Process Control

Measurable Process Control, or SPC, is the method created by Shewhart in 1924. It exists to screen or manage a process to promise its capacities to its most outstanding abilities.

SPC is a method of value control utilizing insights. If the process continues as before, the result will continue as before; you can anticipate what will occur later on, depending on what happened previously. Through his SPC ideas, Shewhart uncovered that having a production process in a condition of measurable control and keeping it in factual control was necessary to foresee the future yield from a particular production process.

In SPC, rather than adjusting issues after they happen, there is an accentuation on early disclosure and shirking of issues. This method makes it less likely that a finished item should be changed.

Fundamental Phases of Activity in Statistical Process Control:

* Comprehend a process
* Understand the determination furthest reaches of the process
* Make the process stable by evacuating assignable, unordinary reasons for variety.
* Detect critical changes of mean or variety by observing the continuous production process. Use control graphs as an apparatus to screen a process.

To actualize factual process control, Shewhart joins the idea of measurable power with the utilization of control graphs.

Control Charts

Created in 1924, Shewhart's control outline was otherwise called Shewhart's Charts, process conduct diagrams, and as control graphs. Control graphs are tools utilized in factual process control. These graphs are used to finish up whether a business process or manufacturing process is now in a condition of accurate control.

When a control graph shows that a process is steady or leveled out (where the main varieties are set up by types that are regular to the process), no changes are required for the operation. The outline would now be able to be utilized to estimate the future yield of this process.

When a controlled outline shows that a process is temperamental or not in control, the diagram must be investigated to see where the remarkable variety is originating from. It is imperative to make sense of where the issue is coming from, with the goal that the process's yield isn't upset.

These are found on a control diagram:

- Statistical focuses that speak to estimations of a process's quality characteristics. These accurate estimations of value are recovered from the yield of a process on various occasions so they can be utilized for correlation.
- The mean of accurate estimations of value is recorded by the centerline drawn at this number on the control outline.
- The standard blunder or deviation is determined dependent on the entirety of the accurate estimations of value that were gathered.
- The graph is set apart with lower control cutoff points and upper control cutoff points to indicate the number where the process production is improbable (factually).

William Edwards Deming

In 1927, Deming met with Walter A. Shewhart. Deming was dazzled with Shewhart's ideas of factual process control. W. Edwards Deming, an American who lived from October 14, 1900, to December 20, 1993. Deming was an administration expert, analyst, engineer, creator, speaker, and teacher. Deming contemplated Shewhart's work on measurable control, control outlines, and Shewhart's straight-line process. Shewhart's idea of underlying reasons for variety (known, memorable, having to do with the process, and quantifiable) and different reasons for type (measurable varieties that are obscure/haven't occurred previously, irregular unquantifiable) legitimately prompted Deming's hypothesis of the executives. Deming perceived that Shewhart's ideas and processes could be applied to manufacturing processes and the processes that oversee organizations.

Deming altered a four-section arrangement of talks that Shewhart gave in 1937. These talks were distributed in a 1939 book called Statistical Method from the Viewpoint of Quality Control. During the 1930s in the US, Deming worked with the US Census Bureau to help build up the inspecting strategies they utilized in 1940 and still today. In 1943, Deming instructed engineers and extra individuals (on the side of war endeavors) in his first seminar on essential applied insights. At that point, Deming started a multi-year showing program, encouraging the measurement training program at Stanford. Deming.org says that here he taught near 2000 individuals on the PDSA Cycle and the Shewhart Cycle for Learning and Improvement.

Deming went on, in 1950, to encourage individuals about ideas of value and factual process control (SPC). In Japan, Deming showed several top administration industrialists, researchers, designers, and directors. Deming's principle instructing to officials was that expanded quality abatements use and build efficiency and piece of the pie. Different manufacturers in Japan followed Deming's strategies to accomplish new degrees of efficiency and quality. Another global interest for items originating from Japan emerged because of their diminished expense and expanded quality. During the 1950s, from the processes dependent on what Deming educated, Japan was on the way to turning into the world's second-biggest economy. Deming can be credited for carrying the possibility of continuous improvement to Japan.

Training Within Industry (TWI)

TWI was run within a US government organization, the War Manpower Commission, from the year 1940 through 1945. This program was set up as a crisis administration in the US during World War II. The United States Government War Production Board made TWI.

From the industry, specialists were drafted to create methods to accelerate war materials production quickly. The program was expected to prepare new untalented workers in the war production workforce rapidly. These new workers were expected to supplant the talented workforce (that were delivering war materials) that was presently taking off to war.

The TWI programs comprised of first training meetings: they were separated into four projects that were every 10 hours in length. The TWI program was created by Charles R. Allen's 4 stage method of training new workers: Show, Tell, Do Check. Charles R. Allen was a Massachusetts professional educator. In 1917, during World War I, Charles was designated to head a program to increment prepared workers for the boat building industry 10-overlap.

The Four TWI training programs:

- Job Instruction (JI): The course was to show experienced workers, directors, and chiefs to prepare undeveloped representatives rapidly. Mentors appeared to take jobs and separate them into small-characterized ventures to exhibit the means while clarifying the fundamental advances and their purpose. And afterward, to intently watch the understudy show the system, mentor them, and gradually end instructing as the understudy can do it without the coach.

- Job Methods (JM): This was a course to instruct workers to assess (impartially) the job's effectiveness fastidiously and recommend consistent improvements. If the worker thought of a wasteful undertaking, they were accused of the errand of thinking of an answer by disposing of something, joining steps, improving, or disentangling steps. The worker should then present the plan to coworkers and their director and attempt to pick up endorsement.
- Job Relations (JR): This course was to show chiefs/managers to deal with representatives both successfully and in a reasonable way.
- Program Development (PD): This was a meeting to instruct mentors to help tackle tackling issues of production through intense training.

The Economic and Scientific Section (ESS) bunch was relegated to improving Japan's administration abilities after WWII. Some portion of their work was to encourage the Training Within Industry programs in Japan appropriately. To help in their work, ESS presented a TWI training film. This TWI training film showed Job Instruction (JI), Job Methods (JM), and Job Relations (JR). The TWI training film was classified as "Improvement in 4 Steps." In Japanese, this means *Kaizen eno Yon Nankai*. Some consider this to be the proper presentation of Kaizen into Japan. The TWI training was broadly acknowledged in Japan as it and Deming's lessons formed into Kaizen's establishment.

The Toyota Motor Corporation

Toyota Motor Corporation was one of the organizations that saddled the information on Kaizen, the lessons of Deming, and the TWI program in Japan. In 1950, Toyota set up utilizing quality circles. Deming first depicted quality circles before that year. They are otherwise called quality control circles. A quality circle can be characterized as gatherings of representatives with a similar job or the same job who get together reliably to describe, examine, and offer answers for issues identified with their work. A director regularly heads the gathering. This administrator will, at that point, carry the arrangements of the meeting to higher administration.

The utilization of value circles and the TWI training programs helped lead to the Toyota Production System's advancement (TPS). The Toyota Production System depends on the way of thinking of the all-out destruction of all waste, or "Muda." The system uses Kaizen, Just-In-Time, and Jidoka. Today, despite everything, Toyota utilizes TPS and devotes time and vitality to impart the system to different businesses.

Taiichi Ohno's Toyota Production System

Businessman and modern designer Taiichi Ohno was the central Japanese business figure to parlay Deming-style quality control into staggering, world-driving outcomes. Ohno began building up the Toyota Production System (TPS) in 1945 and refined it until about 1965. TPS, otherwise called "without a moment to spare" manufacturing, is a system for lessening waste and augmenting efficiencies through continuous improvement. It is additionally recognized as a significant cause of the Lean business procedure.

When it was first formulated, TPS was a last-discard endurance system for the automaker to explore the scraggly after war years. Toyota's future suitability as an organization was flawed. The best-case scenario and assets were rare. A portion of the after-war hardware their plants utilized had been discounted, taken from the garbage pile, and returned to work through a mix of specialized resourcefulness and sheer need. Physically missing, Ohno attempted to make the most elite resources he had—workers with cerebrums and abilities.

Ohno's way of thinking is embodied in his "Ten Commandments" for speculation and winning:

1. Try to eliminate waste and perceive that you are an expense.
2. State "I can do it" and make a decent attempt.
3. The workplace is your educator. You can just discover your answers there.
4. In case you will do anything, do it immediately. The best way to win is to begin now.
5. When you begin something, never surrender. Drive forward until it's done.
6. Fundamentally clarify complex ideas. If a plan is easy to comprehend, rehash it.
7. Bring your problems out away from any detectable hindrance.
8. Understand that actions without esteem are awful.
9. Continue improving profitability and improving what has just been enhanced.
10. Practice and offer wisdom, don't only accumulate it.

Ohno was a hesitant professional chief, who, when all is said in done, liked to be "the place the action is," so he imposed this way of thinking on others in oversight positions. His TPS advanced mindful process permeability, which means checking out the quick and dirty subtleties of actual manufacturing on the factory floor, posing a ton of inquiries, and finding the small, shrouded processes that are disguising a considerable measure of waste.

The TPS system worked well; Toyota developed year on year, and deals went up reliably. By 2008, Toyota outperformed General Motors in worldwide sales, a position GM had been clutching for a long time. TPS was elevated individual to individual by Ohno's mentorship. He trained understudies who became coaches, who shown different understudies, etc. until TPS turned into a pervasive idea within Toyota and spread outwards to other Japanese organizations.

Ohno's innovations (in the end) offered to ascend to the prosaism of Japanese autos that are modest and decline to bite the dust, going from proprietor to proprietor through the span of numerous decades. This is a uber-unmistakable case of how kaizen, as epitomized in TPS and subsidiary systems at other car organizations like Honda, Suzuki, and Nissan, can accomplish emotional outcomes.

Masaaki Imai brings kaizen toward the West and the rest.

Masaaki Imai, a Japanese administration specialist, is practical without any assistance liable for bringing kaizen toward the West. Since the 1960s, he's worked with several remote and joint-adventure organizations inside and outside of Japan. Imai is the smash hit 1986 book Kaizen: The Key to Japan's Competitive Success. He followed that up during the 90s with Gemba Kaizen: A Commonsense, Low-cost Approach to Management (1997). Imai also began the Kaizen Institute (established in 1986), which causes associations to execute kaizen practices within neighborhood social and business practices.

Imai's idea of kaizen is centered on improving and looking after tasks, climbing the field bit by bit instead of gunning for the Hail Mary touchdown play. Expressly, he underlines the "esteem included" part of your business because conveying esteem is everything. Likewise significant for Imai is Gemba, which means the actual spot where the work happens—regardless of whether that be a doctor's office, a shop room floor, or a change over space office space. He accepts chiefs must devote an essential measure of time to Gemba rather than concentrating on the "style" and glory of

R&D and showcasing.

This implies administrators must defeat the verifiable dread of being uncovered as oblivious, investigating the small aspects of business, and asking what may appear to be necessary inquiries.

In Kaizen: The Key to Japan's Competitive Success, Imai noticed how Japan's organizations were process-situated, thus, on a fundamental level, contradicted America's outcomes arranged culture. Separating Japan's achievement in quality control and improvement, he found that process-arranged reasoning advances straightforwardness, and all-encompassing systems see that isn't one-sided via "carrot and stick" thinking. Japan had gained notoriety for inexpensively "not very good" items during the 1950s and 1960s. However, with kaizen principles applied year-on-year at significant firms, the nation's things transformed consistently towards notoriety for reliable high caliber by the 1980s.

The way of thinking was supported up by the consequences of a kaizen venture the board at significant Japanese firms like Fuji-Xerox, Toyota, Canon, and Honda, which by the 1980s reliably beat their American partners. American industry followed through on a dear cost for not focusing on Deming at home. At that point, in 1980, NBC broadcast 60 minutes in length section called "If Japan Can, Why Can't We?" seen by millions, acquainting numerous Americans with Deming. In 1981, he was employed by Ford, who was battling with $3 billion in misfortunes in 3 years and fundamentally spared the organization. In 1987, President Reagan gave him the National Medal of Technology.

Deming's lessons had returned stateside and encouraged a financial rebound. In 1997, the Lean Enterprise Institute was established, bringing Deming's thoughts into new zones.

Kaizen practices are setting explicit.

"Kaizen develops exceptionally within every association, following changes to the association's business condition. Nitty-gritty usage shifts significantly. Kaizen is a way of thinking that produces better long-haul results, an approach to continuously improve gradually. Indeed, the story of the Tortoise and the Hare discovers contemporary significance. It's in every case more financially savvy to work on holding the clients you as of now have, as opposed to go out and attempt to win new ones. Additionally, kaizen's strategy commenced on tweaking your current resource base to convey better execution, spares you the time, expenses, and potential blowback of a sensational upgrade.

On a fundamental level, to appropriately coordinate kaizen practices into your business, you should document your standardized work processes through a bit by bit approach that shows your workflow. For this, a kanban board or other straightforward work representation apparatus will do pleasantly. In the meantime, individuals in authority positions need to establish corporate culture's pace by acting as they'd like every other person to respond. Setting high close to home and gathering conduct standards advances an environment of transparency.

Since individuals are persuaded by encouraging feedback, it is essential to cultivate a culture of inborn motivating forces. This should also be clarified starting from the top (regardless of whether your association is a small gathering without a reasonable chain of importance). Your colleagues ought to be happy to make recommendations; however, they need to because they feel esteemed, and therefore actually put resources into the organization's progress.

While kaizen can be a remunerating process all by itself, it turns out to be genuinely self-supporting when colleagues consider the investment to be mirroring their circumstances. That implies kaizen should be worked around taking care of problems that are fulfilling to unravel and as an outcome support spirit. These problems will involve anything from process refinement to item improvement to principal workplace issues. This is precarious, to a point, because kaizen works best when your goals are humble. For a large portion of us, modest does not ordinarily equivalent fervor, yet long haul improvement should be estimated to forestall significant, bogus advances.

In Africa, for instance, kaizen approaches are being applied to accomplish little, however economical, innovative triumphs without "big blast" thoughts. Instead of an attempt to contend with the big-spend R&D of financially endowed Western and East Asian partners, African organizations are looking to adjust existing innovation to explain one of a kind nearby issues. By encouraging a business culture of learning, African organizations would like to build neighborhood profitability and accordingly improve nearby government assistance.

Concerning the present item improvement game, speed is a fundamental resource in the mission to endure an inexorably severe condition. Kaizen, with its transient innovation cycles outfitted towards long haul success, is appropriate to say business as usual. An approach to escaping the Crisis and into a definite benefit, kaizen gives the establishment to contending in an inexorably mind-boggling condition by slicing through the layers of system-building, finding true worth and afterward removing waste. It's an exceptionally human method for running a system, placing confidence in your group fair and square of the person. Also, we people truly do perspire the easily overlooked details, so why not put resources into consummating them?

CHAPTER TWO

WHY KAIZEN IS EFFECTIVE

How Kaizen works

The accomplishment of Kaizen lies in the contribution of all representatives at each degree of an organization. As opposed to a top-down or base-up approach, each individual is urged to share proposals for improvements. Through the aggregate individual endeavors of a whole association, small improvements can be actioned over each business zone to accomplish continuous innovation – after some time, having a vast by and significant effect. Furthermore, engaging representatives to have a state on workplace changes supports assurance, which, like this, prompts higher profitability levels.

What's the distinction between Kaizen and innovation?

Kaizen's critical contrast and innovation are that Kaizen is a continuous process, while change can be considered a progressively extreme action. Kaizen centers around small improvements that can be effectively taken on a standard and steady premise to convey gradual improvements on a long-haul scale. Innovation, then again, centers around enormous, emotional advancements that require speculation and planning, which expect to send critical developments in a moderately short timescale after usage.

How Kaizen and innovation work together

New, new, and inventive thoughts that achieve business improvements are at the focal point of both Kaizen and innovation activities. Through radical changes, an association can give critical improvements in profitability and productivity. In contrast, continuous improvements keep up the force and further expand upon the underlying inventive execution's achievement and advantages.

Both Kaizen and innovation may be active with the contribution and duty of top administration to keep up the energy and focal point of activities. Time and interest in training workers in new processes, strategies, and practices will require responsibility and long haul vision, which administrative changes could endanger. Moreover, without this help, new thoughts could be inadvertently disheartened.

How is Kaizen utilized in coordination?

Supply chains have developed in both multifaceted nature and complexity. In the present interconnected world, various partners across global districts all have a crucial influence. The Kaizen model gives a way to enhance processes without risking the general activity. This is because changes are small and comfortable with moment results. Kaizen's fundamental principles include distinguishing snappy win answers for problems to improve the general standard of the activity and with the full association. Within coordinations, the advantages of Kaizen include:

- Improved job satisfaction
- Better correspondence
- Improved administration and item quality
- Reduction of waste
- Improved intensity
- Improved productivity
- Higher consumer loyalty

Instances of Kaizen in coordination and supply chains can be found in associations over the world. Kaizen structures one of The Toyota Production System's center principles, enabling individual workers to recognize regions for improvement and propose practical arrangements. For

Nestlé, Kaizen has brought about immense improvements in the decrease of waste by bringing down the time and materials on their processes. Here at Yusen Logistics, Kaizen is a piece of the association culture – bolstered by top administration and supported through yearly honors on a local and worldwide scale.

Kaizen best practices

Over the late years, the Kaizen theory has been generally acknowledged across numerous divisions everywhere throughout the world – especially in the production and dissemination businesses – and today is one of the center principles in lean inventory network the executive's frameworks. Following Kaizen best practices will ensure you're continually achieving the most from your drives:

- Ask why
- Solve it together
- Reflect on progress
- Measure execution
- Go to Gemba
- Treat the reason
- Everyone ought to be included

Plan-Do-Check-Act Process

What Is PDCA?

PDCA, now and then called PDSA, the "Deming Wheel," or "Deming Cycle," was created by prestigious administration advisor Dr. William Edwards Deming during the 1950s. Deming himself considered it the "Shewhart Cycle," as his model depended on a thought from his tutor, Walter Shewhart. Deming needed to make a method for recognizing what made items neglect to live up to clients' desires. His answer causes businesses to create speculations about what requirements to change and test them in a continuous criticism circle.

Deming utilized the idea of Plan-Do-Study-Act (PDSA). He found that the attention on Check is progressively about the usage of a change. Deming emphasizes an improvement exertion's consequences, considering the actual outcomes and contrasting them with conceivably reexamine the hypothesis. He focused on that a belief continuously guides the need to grow new information from learning. PDCA/PDSA is an iterative, four-arrange approach for consistently improving processes, items or administrations, and settling problems. It includes systematically testing potential arrangements, evaluating the outcomes, and executing those that are appeared to work.

The four stages are:

- Plan: recognize and examine the problem or opportunity, create theories about what the issues might be, and choose which one to test.
- Do: test the potential arrangement in a perfect world for a small scope and measure the outcomes.
- Check/Study: study the outcome, measure adequacy, and choose whether the speculation is upheld or not.
- Act: if the arrangement was fruitful, actualize it.

The PDCA or PDSA Cycle

The PDCA cycle causes you to take care of problems and actualize arrangements in a thorough, systematic way. Follow these four stages to guarantee that you get the most excellent outcomes.

1. Plan

You have to recognize and comprehend your problem or the

open door that you need to exploit in the first place. Utilizing the initial six stages of The Simplex Process can assist you with doing this by managing you through a process of investigating data, characterizing your problem, producing and screening thoughts, and building up an execution plan.

At the last piece of this stage, state quantitatively what your desires are, if the thought is fruitful, and your problem is settled. You'll come back to this in the Check organize. Before you proceed onward to the following stage, consider utilizing Impact Analysis or ORAPAPA to detect check your plan. You may spot critical problems with it, and it might merit returning to the planning stage.

2. Do

When you've recognized a potential arrangement, test it with a small-scale pilot venture. This will permit you to evaluate whether your proposed changes accomplish the ideal result, with negligible interruption to your activity's reminder if they don't. For instance, you could compose a preliminary within a division, a constrained topographical zone, or a specific segment.

As you run the pilot venture, assemble information to show whether the change has worked or not. You'll utilize this in the following stage. Recall that, right now, signifies "attempt" or "test." It doesn't mean "actualize completely," which occurs at the Act arrange.

3. Check

At this stage, you dissect your pilot undertaking's outcomes against the desires that you characterized in Step 1 to evaluate whether the thought has worked or not. If it hasn't worked, you come back to Step 1. If it has worked, you proceed to Step 4.

You may choose to evaluate more changes and rehash the Do and Check stages – don't agree to a not precisely satisfactory arrangement. Proceed onward to the last step (Act) just when you're genuinely content with the preliminary's results. Deming's model was adjusted during the 1980s by quality administration pioneer Kaoru Ishikawa. As it may, Deming separated himself from these changes and altered his original model during the 1990s. He underscored the significance of study and learning in the third stage. As we featured before, this is the reason the model is, in some cases, alluded to as Plan-Do-Study-Act (PDSA).

4. Act

This is the place you actualize your answer. In any case, recall that PDCA/PDSA is a circle, not a process with a start and an end. This implies your improved process or item turns into the new gauge, and you keep on searching for approaches to make it surprisingly better for your association or clients.

When to Use PDCA/PDSA

The PDCA/PDSA framework can improve any process or item by breaking it into smaller advances. It is especially successful for:

- Helping to actualize Total Quality Management or Six Sigma activities, and for the most part, assisting with improving processes.
- Exploring a scope of answers for problems and guiding them in a controlled path before choosing one for usage.
- I am avoiding wastage of assets by revealing an incapable arrangement on a full scale.

You can utilize the model in a wide range of business situations, from the new item advancement, task, and change the executives, to item lifecycle and production network the board. PDCA is regularly utilized as a framework for executing Kaizen, another system for continuously tweaking your items and processes that underscores the significance of taking out the waste.

The Pros and Cons of PDCA/PDSA

The model is a basic yet fantastic approach to determine new and repeating issues in any industry, division, or process. Its iterative methodology permits you and your group to test arrangements and evaluate brings about a waste-decreasing cycle. It ingrains a pledge to continuous improvement, anyway small, and can improve effectiveness and efficiency in a controlled manner, without the dangers of making enormous scope, untested changes to your processes.

In any case, experiencing the PDCA/PDSA cycle can be much slower than a direct, "gung ho" usage. In this way, it probably won't be a suitable methodology for managing a pressing problem or crisis. It also requires critical "purchase in" from colleagues and offers fewer open doors for radical innovation if that is what your association needs. There are continuous improvement models like PDCA/PDSA, such as Build-Measure-Learn, the After Action Review Process, and The Hoshin Planning System.

This fuses a portion of the principles of PDCA/PDSA; however, they are not substitutes for it. The PDCA/PDSA cycle is a continuous circle of planning, doing, checking (or examining), and acting. It gives a necessary and compelling methodology for taking care of problems and overseeing change. It's helpful for testing improvement gauges for a small scope before refreshing strategies and working methods.

You can utilize it in a wide range of business processes, from growing new items to dealing with the inventory network. The methodology starts with a Planning stage in which problems are unmistakably recognized and comprehended, and measured speculation is created. Potential arrangements are tried for a small scope in the Do stage, and the result is then assessed and checked. You can experience the Do and Check arranges the same number of times as vital before the full, cleaned arrangement is actualized in the Act stage.

Apply This to Your Life:

While PDCA/PDSA is a viable device for businesses, you can likewise utilize it to improve your exhibition. Distinguish what is keeping you down in your profession and how you need to advance. Take a gander at the underlying driver of any issue, and set goals to defeat these deterrents (Plan). At the point when you've settled on your game-plan, test various ways to deal with getting the outcomes that you need (Do). Review progress routinely, change your conduct as needs and think about your actions' consequences (Check). At long last, actualize what's working and ceaselessly refine what isn't (Act).

Distinguishing problems

The craft of problem unraveling is continually attempting to advance and be re-marked by people in different enterprises. At the same time, the new way might just be a successful method in specific applications. A dependable method for recognizing and tackling problems is the eight stages to possible problem unraveling created by Toyota years back. The system is organized yet straightforward and practical enough to deal with the minor nature issues to the most challenging problems.

Utilizing an essential and critical approach to problems makes consistency within an association when you base your outcomes on facts, experience, sound judgment, the issue's structure objective and practically.

The Eight-Step Problem Solving Process

1. Clarify the Problem
2. Breakdown the Problem
3. Set the Target
4. Analyze the Root Cause
5. Develop Countermeasures
6. Implement Countermeasures
7. Monitor Results and Process
8. Standardize and Share Success

The eight stages to practical problem understanding additionally incorporate the (PDCA) cycle. The doing is found in stage six. Stage seven is checking. Phase eight includes acting out the consequences of the new standard.

This practical problem unraveling can be a fantastic asset to issues confronting your association. It permits associations to have a typical comprehension of what characterizes a problem and what steps will be taken to defeat the problem effectively.

The Eight Steps Broken Down:

Stage 1: Clarify the Problem

A problem can be characterized in one of three different ways. The first being, whatever is a deviation from the standard. The second could be the hole between the actual condition and the ideal condition, with the third being an unfilled client need.

To best explain the problem, you need to see the problem with your own eyes. This gives you the subtleties and hands-on experience that will permit you to push ahead in the process.

Stage 2: Breakdown the Problem

When you've seen the problem directly, you can start to breakdown the question into progressively specific and explicit issues. Keep in mind that you, despite everything, need to see the smaller, single issues with your own eyes as you analyze your problem. This is also a decent time to examine and break down the various information sources and yields to organize your endeavors successfully. It is substantially more successful in overseeing and taking care of many miniaturized scale problems, each in turn, as opposed to attempting to handle a big problem with no bearing.

Stage 3: Set the Target

Stage three is about duty and core interest. Your consideration should now concentrate on what is expected to finish the extent and how long it would take to wrap up. You should set focuses on testing, yet within limits, and don't strain the association that would impede the improvement process.

Stage 4: Analyze the Root Cause

This was an essential advance when a problem was illuminating because it will help you distinguish the actual factors that caused the issue in any case. As a general rule, there are numerous main drivers to investigate. Ensure you are thinking about all potential main drivers and tending to them appropriately. Again, an appropriate underlying driver examination includes you setting off to the reason itself rather than depending on reports.

Stage 5: Develop Countermeasures

When you've built up your main drivers, you can utilize that data to build up the countermeasures expected to expel the underlying drivers. Your group ought to create the same number of countermeasures expected to address all underlying drivers legitimately. When you've built up your countermeasures, you can start to limit them down to the most practical and successful based on your objective.

Stage 6: Implement Countermeasures

Since you have built up your countermeasures and limited them down, the time has come to oversee them conveniently. Correspondence is critical in stage six. You'll need to look for thoughts from the group and keep working back through the PDCA cycle to guarantee nothing is being missed en route. Consider executing each countermeasure in turn to screen the adequacy of each. You will indeed commit errors all through your problem illuminating processes. However, your determination is vital, particularly in stage six.

Stage 7: Monitor Results and Process

As missteps occur and countermeasures come up short, you need a system set up to review and alter them to get the planned outcome. You can likewise decide whether the expected result was the consequence of the countermeasure's action, or was it only an accident? There are consistently lots of opportunities to get better in the problem illuminating process, yet you should have the option to remember it regarding your consideration.

Stage 8: Standardize and Share Success

Since you've experienced accomplishment along your problem settling way, the time has come to set the new processes within the association and offer them all through the association. It is additionally a decent time to think about what you've realized and address any potential uncertain issues or inconveniences you have en route. Overlooking unclear effects will just prompt more problems down the street.

At long last, since you are a genuine Lean association that accepts continuous improvement never stops, the time has come to handle the following problem. Start the problem understanding process over again and keep on working towards flawlessness.

Setting New Standards and a Focused Mindset

Current Mindset versus Kaizen Mindset

While executing Kaizen, numerous people center around individuals and process improvement tools and methods, yet they disregard the need to build up a kaizen mindset. This isn't right because kaizen isn't only a device for achieving continuous improvement. It a mindset change – a perspective and doing things. This article talks about the essential aspects of the kaizen mindset.

Kaizen originates from the base.

If you imagine that Kaizen will be business, of course – where the executives will gauge the benefits of every thought – at that point, you are in for a colossal disappointment. Adoption of Kaizen is best when ideas and plans originate from the base up, not top-down. Just those in the actual workstation - doing the assignment - genuinely see precisely what works or what doesn't work for them – the board doesn't have such private presentation. Techniques for improvement originating from them don't prompt functional enhancements.

For instance, in Toyota, during vehicle gathering, they have a pushcart loaded up with all tools they require for this specific job masterminded systematically: no more, no less. The thought is to reduce development just as the time needed for workers to discover tools, thus boosting effectiveness. The theory originated from factory representatives on the floor, who comprehended their agony and what should have been improved to make their work increasingly useful and progressively agreeable.

In this way, allow everybody in your association to propose improvement thoughts.

Kaizen is about change.

If you state that you need to change for the better on the one hand, however, on the other one, you believe that change isn't essential, you should stop Kaizen right away.

Being a Japanese word, Kaizen implies steady or continuous improvement, and any development includes change. In any case, note that kaizen ought not to be executed in a prevailing fashion, it's a long haul system, and the objective is to move towards gradual improvements, which together mean radical successes.

Kaizen is about freedom.

Kaizen isn't tied in with getting authorization to make changes – it is tied in with enabling workers to change things for the better all along. Representatives need to have the freedom to test and to take fundamental actions to improve things. The biggest mix-up that a firm can make is formalizing Kaizen with the end goal that completing jobs becomes bureaucratic and an issue. For instance, Google gave a 20 percent time thought, which prescribes that each worker should invest energy inside ventures once per week. For the most part, they have a field day where they are urged to create thoughts on how they can improve their workplace.

Kaizen is a continuous duty.

Kaizen is a continuous process that never closes. It is the quest for flawlessness. For the most part, it is challenging to accomplish flawlessness: you can generally improve things, so Kaizen should be in a hurry at some random time.

Kaizen includes committing errors.

In Western reasoning, tragically, ruins are generally treated as motivation to teach and rebuff the doer. In Kaizen and Japanese thinking, botches are viewed as a positive thing – something to gain from.

For instance, in a western association, a SMALL Mistake regularly prompts a visit with (risk from) THE Boss and even rejection or disciplinary action. In Toyota, a slip-up frequently prompts directing a careful 5-whys investigation to decide the essential drivers of the problem and create answers to keep it from happening once more. In America, the worker would lose the job. In Japan or Toyota, the worker would improve the position. The Japanese consider this to be an opportunity to grow. If you threaten or fire the worker who knows where he/she failed, what expectation would you need to forestall the reappearance of a similar misstep?

Kaizen's mindset utilizes an experimentation principle. Nothing is excellent, and a large portion of the occasions many refinements should be adopted before an improvement is acknowledged and copied to different divisions. A Kaizen Mindset Leader empowers this principle, while a Current Mindset Manager does not chance the experimentation method.

Kaizen Leadership Mindset

Living the over five focuses will assist pioneers with adopting the Kaizen Mindset. In any case, right now, I will learn six characteristics that draw out the best Kaizen Leadership Mindset.

1. Consistently improvement – A day ought not to go without some type of development being executed someplace in the association.
2. Client driven improvement – Any Kaizen venture should bring about expanded customer satisfaction.
3. Quality first, benefit follows – Organizations can flourish just if their customers are fulfilled.
4. Problems are all over the place – Realization that all associations have issues and set up an association culture where a representative can unreservedly concede these issues and propose arrangements is the ideal approach to execute Kaizen.
5. Problem-taking care of – Problem fathoming ought to be viewed as a synergistic methodology and a cross-useful system.
6. Accentuation on the process – Developing an administration approach that supports process-based endeavors for improvement is vital.

Kaizen Mindset is about continuous improvement, just as making progress toward a condition of flawlessness, where all action makes an incentive for residents and clients. Total flawlessness can't be gotten, yet the Kaizen-thinking associations continually scan for approaches to do things better.

They attempt to reduce waste, making them less ready to understand their goals and utilize their restricted assets in manners that do not prompt the company's general purposes. As you will see underneath, there are various sorts of waste that influence an association.

Fruitful Implementation of Kaizen

These are the things that all supervisors ought to get ready to make kaizen execution a smooth encounter.

Be prepared for obstruction.

Individuals lean toward the state of affairs – they dislike changing the standards. As indicated by an investigation directed by the Lean Enterprise Institute or LEI, an administration inquire about firm protections, particularly from the central administration, is the main hindrance to actualizing Kaizen.

38% of the respondents to this yearly examination about business system usage set the top reason for kaizen disappointment in central administration, trailed by the absence of ability at 31%, and representatives' opposition at 27.7%. This was as opposed to the earlier year (2014) review that referred to losing the faith as the number reason for the absence of improvement, trailed by the lack of expertise, and afterward, center administration opposition.

I was right doing and training.

All representatives ought to be all around prepared to eliminate struggle and convey a gathering that can encourage significant improvement. This implies learning by doing first and afterward training later.

For instance, the Toyota system consistently prescribes its representatives to learn by doing things. In the beginning times of Kaizen usage, the firm prescribes 80 percent doing and 20 percent training just as data. Their system includes placing the representatives in various circumstances and letting them create answers for multiple problems.

Expand on association's foundations

Toyota has a remarkable way. Associations need to have one-of-a-kind ways as well. For example, when Toyota works with associations to educate TPS, they generally demand that the associations build up their systems. Somebody accomplished something effectively to get your association to this point. Expand on that. Enhance your association's legacy to distinguish a big motivator for you.

Training your mind to acknowledge the change

Small advances

Initially, we center on applying these "small advances," the soul of Kaizen reasoning. Recall those small goals lead to more rewards. If your goals are low, at that point, everything will be more straightforward. Your cerebrum will believe 'it's overly simple' I realize how to do it, fantastic! Presently it's the ideal opportunity for action, so don't hesitate. Pick one small objective every day that will assist you with developing yourself efficiently.

If you are somebody who needs to deal with your body, however consistently discovers pardons not to, reveal to yourself one of these:

– I will do five sit-ups in the first part of the day in the wake of awakening, or – I will do five crunches in the first part of the day after awakening, or – I will eat one spoon of rice/noodles/or a chomp of pizza short of what I used to. If you need to expand your insight and become more intelligent, reveal to yourself one of these:

– I'll peruse a passage consistently from the reference book, or – I'll read one page of highbrow writing a day. If you need to become familiar with another dialect:

– I'll learn a new word per day, or – I'll discover and record one sentence in a language that I need to become familiar with consistently. If you need to stop smoking:

– I will discard one cigarette daily rather than dragging it. If you feel discouraged and desolate:

– Once every day for 2 minutes, I will consider some lovely minute I imparted to somebody near me. If you imagine that sitting the entire day before the PC is harming your wellbeing:

– Once every day, I will stand up alongside my work area and stretch for a moment, or – I will get off the transport one-stop prior and walk home.

These goals are little to such an extent that they sound strange. However, it truly works ponders sooner or later. At the point when you become acclimated to them and increment your exertion, you won't notice that you have.

Small Questions Method

Another Kaizen strategy, which we can without much of a stretch apply to regular day-to-day existence, is the "small inquiries" method. Each clinician concurs that asking yourself inquiries is more propelling than guiding yourself. For instance, If you go out on the town to shop for staple goods, rather than letting you know: "presently I need to purchase something solid," ask yourself an inquiry: "what sound nourishment would I be able to buy here? Right now, the fact of the matter is to program your mind into deduction: how might I make myself more advantageous? - Rather than regarding it as a commitment. The equivalent could apply to work out. Rather than letting yourself know: "I should run more!" figure: "how might I be increasingly fit?" This sort of addressing is significantly more stimulating than merely driving yourself to do something.

Deal with the Small Things Quickly

Everybody attempts to stay away from obligations now and again. Any individual who has numerous commitments realizes that it is so critical to managing them steadily. The small things look so honest that we will, in general, overlook them until they heap up and get hard to manage rapidly. If you need to react to a message – do it immediately. It might take two or three minutes to respond, yet make a stab at responding to 15 words that have accumulated. It devours a great deal of vitality superfluously! You should have a go at giving yourself 2 minutes. Make it a rule – if something takes under 120 seconds, I will do it right away!

If you need to change your life, you need to begin today and remain with it consistently. There are no exceptional cases. Always you are going to gain some small ground without seeing it. You will discover that following seven days, a month, a year, two years, that there has been a tremendous change, your advancement has been gigantic! The means are little to such an extent that you can't fizzle.

CHAPTER THREE

THE IMPORTANCE OF HAVING HABITS AND WHY IT IS SO HARD TO CHANGE THEM

Why habits are significant

Habits can be incredibly helpful, and it is challenging to run our lives without them. They robotize many of the usual activities in our lives and let loose our minds, so we are fit for focusing on more elevated level activities.

For instance, if we needed to deliberately consider essential capacities like strolling orbiting our nourishment or talking, we would have no psychological ability accessible to perform different functions. The capacity to compose or type naturally permits us to concentrate on delivering an excellent article, letter, email, or novel. Additionally, strolling via programmed processes allows us to have the option to consider where we are going! We have a considerable number of these vast 'habits' that our muscle memory has developed after some time. In any event, breathing can be thought of as a profoundly instilled habit. Driving a vehicle and riding a bicycle are all of the progressions of practices and actions we perform without a conscious plan.

Along these lines, habits assume a significant job in rearranging our lives and REDUCING the measure of sensory upgrades we have to process. It's evaluated that out of each 11,000 signs we get from our faculties, our mind just intentionally processes 40. Habits spare us vitality as by their tendency, they are programmed and require minimal physical and mental quality; for example, brushing your teeth or tying your shoelaces requires next to no psychological vitality.

Great habits serve to make schedule, request, and effectiveness. Sadly unfortunate propensities have the contrary impact and can secure us in cynical or inflexible examples of conduct. For instance, poor habits, such as gorging, smoking, or driving too quickly, can harm our well-being and prosperity. Our cerebrums are incredibly amazing and are continually filtering for designs in our lives or things it can transform into habits. Sadly, our subliminal mind does not segregate among significant and negative behavior patterns, and anything that is rehashed after some time can turn into a practice.

Luckily, we can assume responsibility for this process and deliberately pick which considerations, actions, and practices will become habits.

The Importance of Habits and How to Build Them

Your habits assume a significant job in your life. Having great habits will lead you to a viable entity. Having unfortunate propensities, then again, will lead you to disappointments. So you must assemble great patterns. Scott Adams once said that "Washouts have goals and victors have systems." But what systems do you have to have? I accept that one of them is a habit-building system. The explanation? Since great habits don't occur naturally.

The fact is: we will, in general, pick the easy way. We will, in general, follow the easy way out. Composing, for example, doesn't come effectively for me. If I didn't have a system for doing it, days or even weeks could pass by without me composing. I needed to manufacture the habit.

Here are a few hints on building habits:

1. Be Balanced

It's critical to carry on with a healthy lifestyle. Regarding habit-building, that implies you should assemble habits in each of the five aspects of life. Building habits in only a couple of issues (for example, Work). However, disregarding the others (for example, Health) will mess up your life in the long haul.

2. Start Small

In building new habits, start small. You can begin with a lower than usual practice. What's significant isn't the amount you do it; however, how predictable you do it.

3. Utilize a Tool

It will be simpler for you to fabricate habits if you have an instrument to assist you with doing it. For my situation, I use Habit Master. It gives me checklists of my day-by-day, weekly, and month-to-month habits. I should simply work through the rundowns, and I realize that I'll be acceptable.

4. Pick Carefully

A significant piece of habit-building is picking what habits to assemble. Your assets are restricted, so you should be cautious in choosing what habits to construct. Pick just the ones that can have the most effect in your life.

5. Assemble Just a Few at Once

A common purpose behind disappointment in habit building is to fabricate such a large number of habits on the double. It transpired. I once had a not insignificant rundown of patterns to assemble. Furthermore, what was the deal? I got focused on it. I got depleted before the days over. After a short time, I simply quit doing them out and out!

So assemble only a couple of habits without a moment's delay. The watchword here is a need.

6. Observe Victories

You have to have a critical system that can give you a feeling of achievement If you do well. This is critical to keep you propelled over the long haul.

For my situation, it gives me a feeling of achievement to see my checklists completely set apart in Habit Master. It lets me state to myself, "I did it!"

7. Expand upon What You've Built

When you have fabricated some healthy habits, you can expand on them. How? By doing to a greater extent, a pattern or building another practice identified with it.

For example, suppose beforehand you focus on perusing books for 30 minutes per day. In that case, you can build it to 45 minutes every day (a more considerable amount of that habit), or you can add tuning in to digital recordings to it (a related new practice). Simply be mindful so as not to overdo it, or you may get worn out. Habits are fundamental for your viability. The significant thing is to be deliberate in building them. Manufacture a system. Focus on it. That is how you can expand your sustainability.

The significance of having solid habits and how to ingrain them in kids

For what reason is it so significant for kids to have solid habits? Healthy habits help youngsters grow upbeat and reliable just as add to forestalling future medical issues, such as diabetes, hypertension, elevated cholesterol, coronary illness, and malignant growth. Hence, we will concentrate on the three mainstays of a healthy lifestyle: a decent eating regimen, physical exercise, and individual cleanliness.

A Balanced Diet

As a factor that impacts the right development and advancement, both honestly and intellectually, kids, a fluctuated and adjusted eating routine are essential. Breakfast is a crucial supporter for kids since it gives them the vitality they need to confront a day loaded with activities. Subsequently, we should perceive what a good breakfast ought to contain. What should a decent breakfast include? A dairy substance (milk, yogurt, new cheddar, and so on.), starches (grains, bread, and so on.), and organic product (original, natural product servings of mixed greens, regular juices, and so on.).

When all is said in done, the accompanying eating regimen arrangements are advised for kids to accomplish great sustenance:

1. More foods are grown from the ground.
2. Less protein.
3. More oats.
4. Less cheap food.

Cleanliness in the eating regimen

Nourishment is continually presented to contamination factors using water, air, soil, ourselves, creatures, and other living creatures, so it is necessary to adhere to essential eating regimen rules of individual cleanliness.

1. Wash your hands before eating any nourishment.
2. Wash products of the soil before eating them.

3.   Drink clean water.
4.   Follow termination dates of nourishment.
5.   Reject protruding, rusted, or harmed holders.

Play sports

An all-around supported youngster has more vitality to learn and build up an adequate physical capacity. Playing sports, at that point, is fundamental for youngsters to grow up cheerful and sound. Today, youngsters are familiar with investing energy, since their bodies should be progressively active, so we should guarantee that our little ones may play sports and spend time outdoors.

How do we ingrain these habits?

We instruct through the model. Ingraining solid habits in our youngsters will prompt both short and long haul improvements in their satisfaction and, accordingly, they will carry on with a more helpful life into adulthood. We can guarantee this more useful life.

1. Presenting each or two habits in turn, it isn't fitting to show all the ideal changes simultaneously. Instead, when these a couple of patterns are absorbed, proceed onward to the accompanying ones.

2. Educating through model; show activities, for example, strolling all together, eating healthy, or washing our hands before eating, and so forth. Taking an interest in these solid habits will show the little ones comprehend that these habits are not disciplines, yet actions of a healthy life that we as a whole do together.

3. Fortifying the habits we need to impart without making tension; eliminate negative expressions, for example, "Do not do this, do not eat that … " and supplanting them with positive ones like "This is flavorful, how about we take a

walk … "

4. Showing the bases of a decent eating regimen eagerly and interactively; remember your kids for suppers' readiness and offer the purposes for your sound decisions.

Why Are Habits Automatic?

In a developmental sense, the automaticity of habits is fundamental to our endurance. Neglectfulness is commonly an element, not a bug. Patterns are what permits us to work on the planet.

If we must be intentionally mindful of the considerable number of a great many miniaturized scale choices we make each day, we could never go anyplace. Envision, we needed to unequivocally gauge the advantages and disadvantages of practices like whether to wash our hands every time we utilized the washroom. Your mind makes up just 2% of your total mass. However, it devours 20% of all the oxygen you breathe in. By need, cerebrums are the most proficient processors on the planet, continually settling on significant tradeoffs between choice quality and choice speed.

Each minimal choice settled on comes to the detriment of choice quality for all our different options. Any decision that can be eliminated opens up intellectual assets that can be diverted towards higher significance choices. Habits adequately permit our cerebrums to redistribute a portion of the snort work of dynamic to our surroundings. As patterns become progressively programmed, neural activity moves from the prefrontal cortex to the basal ganglia. The basal ganglia, probably the most seasoned structure in our mind, is absolved from the process of reasoning. From the mind's viewpoint, this is speculative administrative chemistry for a fantastic scope.

Activated by Context

Habits arise through acquainted learning, most broadly exhibited in Pavlov's trials with dogs. A setting trigger can be anything in our inward or outer condition in which we partner with the habit. Each time a habit is rehashed in a steady setting, our minds fortify the relationship between the practice and the trigger.

The Habit Loop

This carries us to the Habit Loop, an accommodating framework originating in The Power of Habit, which deconstructs a habit into its three-segment parts:

1. Triggers are relevant subtleties which your cerebrum has recently connected with a pattern. Triggers set the habit circle moving by sending our cerebrum into auto-pilot.
2. Behaviors are the actual habit reaction showed. Practices can be either action performed remotely or reactive examples of thought.
3. Rewards fortify a habit, making our mind reinforce the related connection between the Trigger and human behavior.

Triggers, Behaviors, and Rewards are our three potential purposes of influence when we make and fortify our habits. By concentrating on our present habit bottleneck, the "most fragile connection" of the three, we can enormously quicken the habit-building process. In the following three posts, I will tell you the best way to figure out which part of the Habit Loop is your bottleneck and spread out demonstrated procedures for assaulting that powerless connection.

I will close the present prologue to habits with an allegory to help you imagine our general changing practice technique.

Upstream Effects

Close your eyes for a minute. Envision you are water flowing down a waterway. When a watercourse is framed, water hollows out a diversion for itself in the earth. Consistently the water flows, the channel becomes more extensive and more profound. The course the water flows downstream is controlled by the state of a channel framed over numerous years. The waterway can flow an alternate way if the chain is diverted.

Habits work similarly. Each time a pattern is rehashed, our stream channel gets further, as each action makes that action almost sure later on. Our conduct is anticipated by our current natural setting and the habits we have recently connected to that unique circumstance. We can reshape our future behavior by diverting our waterway to another channel [changing our context] or reshaping our chain after some time [linking new habits to that context].

Actions taken to change our habits go before the actual habit change. To divert the waterway, we should go upstream from the planned goal. In this way, I call the actions we take to change our habits upstream impacts. The more drawn out a habit has existed, the more profound the waterway channel will turn into. In this way, it will require relatively more exertion to change. Notwithstanding, when the flow is diverted, all downstream (future) practices will be influenced.

Default Thinking

Think about our habits as our defaults. Each circumstance we wind up in will have a default affiliation and reaction. As our consideration turns out to be progressively rare, it appears to be sheltered to accept that we will gradually default to our defaults. With a concentrated exertion, our defaults can be incidentally be defeated progressively. This exertion is praiseworthy, however impractical. Just salmon have the live programming to go against the flow for such a long time.

If your everyday habits expect control to execute, you're doing it wrong. With a habit-driven methodology, we don't "do things" as much as "make the things we need to do simpler to do later on." Divert that discipline towards building systems that can divert the flow of our future conduct by making your habits simpler to perform. Therefore, habit building is certainly not a one-time exertion; however, a progressing process of perception and rectification of our defaults. It is a learnable meta-aptitude that we practice (or disregard) for the duration of our lives.

"what we more than once do, are We. Greatness at that point, isn't an act, however a habit."— Will Durant. Each action taken is the input we use to reshape our default reaction for comparative circumstances later on. As we approach habit dominance, we recover impact over our conduct, turning out to be creators of our own lives instead of just characters. Nothing we ever do occurs in a vacuum. A treat eaten today reinforces the habit of eating treats, expanding the odds of another gift being eaten tomorrow. The decisions we settle on today decide the decisions that will be made for us tomorrow.

Is It So Hard To Change Habits? - Your Life Goals are Not Your Habits

Your brassy life goals are fantastic. We're pleased with you for having them. In any case, it's conceivable that those goals are intended to distract you from what's genuinely alarming you—the move in everyday habits that would mean a re-innovation of how you see yourself. — Seth Godin

We, as a whole, have expectations and dreams. Also, more often than not, we have, in any event, a general feeling of what those goals are. How we need our bodies to look great and how we appreciate wellbeing, the regard we need to get from our companions and the significant work we need to make, the connections we need with our loved ones, and the affection we need to share.

Generally speaking, this is something worth being thankful for. It's pleasant to recognize what you need, and to have goals provides you with a feeling of guidance and reason. Notwithstanding, there is one way that your deepest desires harm you from getting better: your wants can, without much of a stretch, draw you into taking on more than you could deal with.

You know exactly what I mean.

- You get motivated by The Biggest Loser, head to the rec center, bust your butt to the point of weariness, and take the following three months off to recuperate.
- You, at last, understand that desire to compose your book, arrange the entire day throughout the end of the week, and afterward head back to your regular employment on Monday and never return to it.
- You're roused by your companion's accounts of heading out to new nations, so you begin to plan your own far and wide outing, just to wind up overpowered by all the subtleties and remain at home.

Over and over again, we let our inspirations and wants to drive us into a furor as we attempt to take care of our whole problem without a moment's delay instead of beginning a small, new daily practice.

I know, I know. It's not as attractive as saying you shed 30 pounds in 3 months. In all actuality, this: the fantasies you have are altogether different from the actions that will get you there. So how do we balance our craving to make life-changing changes with the need to assemble small, feasible habits?

Think beyond practical boundaries, But Start Small

In case you're not kidding about rolling out genuine improvement — at the end of the day, If you're not kidding about doing things better than you are currently — you need to begin small. Envision the run of the mill habits, positive or negative: Brushing your teeth and putting your safety belt on, and gnawing your nails. These actions are minute enough for you don't consider them. You do them naturally. They are modest actions that become reliable examples.

Wouldn't it bode well that If we needed to shape new habits, the ideal approach to begin is to roll out little improvements that our cerebrum could rapidly learn and naturally rehash? Imagine a scenario in which you started thinking about your life goals, not as big, nervy things that you can accomplish when all is good and well or when you have better assets or when you at last catch your big break. However, instead of minor, everyday practices are rehashed until progress gets inescapable.

Imagine a scenario where shedding 50 pounds wasn't reliant on a scientist finding the ideal eating regimen or you finding a superhuman dose of resolve, however, it depended on a progression of minor habits that you could generally control. Do some practice like strolling for 20 minutes out of each day, drinking eight glasses of water each day, eating two dinners rather than three.

If you plant the correct seed in the exact spot, it will develop, moving along without any more cajoling. I accept this is the best similitude for making habits. The "right seed" is the modest conduct that you pick. The "urging" part is amping up inspiration, which I think has nothing to do with making habits. Concentrating on motivation as the way to practice is exactly off-base. Leave me alone progressively straightforward: If you pick the correct small conduct and succession it right, at that point, you won't need to rouse yourself to have it develop. It will merely usually happen, similar to a decent seed planted in a suitable spot.

How extraordinary is that?

The regular methodology is to plunge into the deep end when you get a dose of inspiration, just to flop rapidly and wish you had more self-discipline as your new habit suffocates. The new methodology is to swim into the shallow water, gradually going further until you arrive at where you can swim, whether you're inspired or not.

Concentrate on Lifestyle, Not Life–Changing

Again and again, we get fixated on making life–evolving changes.

• Losing about 50 pounds will be life-changing; drinking eight glasses of water every day is another kind of lifestyle.

• Publishing your first book would be life-changing; messaging another book specialist every day is another sort of lifestyle.

• Running a long-distance race would be life-changing; running three days of the week is another kind of lifestyle.

• Earning an extra $20,000 every year would be life-changing; working an additional 5 hours of the week as a specialist is another kind of lifestyle.

• Squatting 100 additional pounds would be life-changing; hunching down three days of the week is another kind of lifestyle.

Do you see the distinction?

Life goals are a great idea to have because they give guidance. However, they can likewise fool you into taking on beyond what you can deal with. Everyday habits — little schedules that are repeatable — are what make big dreams a reality.

Why are habits so difficult to break? - Addiction, Model-Free Learning, and Reward Devaluation

Substance use has frequently been depicted as "terrible learning" connected with disabilities in remuneration processing and dynamic. However, there is minimal considerable research to help this thought. Byrne et al. recommend that substance abuse not just advances hurtful habit development, which may undermine endurance, yet also makes it hard to quit utilizing.

Without model versus Model-based Learning

The "Double Systems" hypothesis of support learning characterizes two unmistakable systems:

1. The model-based, or objective coordinated system, where actions are planned and deliberate, we find out about the association among actions and results and how to change our conduct to accomplish the ideal outcome. This system requires increasingly subjective processing and is progressively adaptable

and controlled.

2. Without a model or habit-based system, reflexive reactions educate learning to improvements - like enthusiastic substance use and yearnings. This system of learning is less adaptable and is increasingly controlled via programmed processing.

The contrasts between the two learning systems have been featured by analysts comparable to unsafe habitual practices, for example, substance use. One way of thinking proposes that education educated by the sans model system, with all the more emphasis on instinctual reaction to improvements and lesser degree attention on informed and educated dynamics, sets an individual up to be bound to take part in harmful practices like substance use.

Substance Use and Reward Devaluation

Prize cheapening is a process that happens in the cerebrum where the estimation of an alluring result, such as singing in a band, tutoring, or keeping up the balance, is reduced altogether. This process plays into why improving treatment results can be so tricky - fixation treatment isn't as "strengthening" in mind as substance use. Enthusiastic medication use is considered "profoundly pleasurable" by the cerebrum pieces that control dynamic when individuals are vigorously dependent and feel just as they need the substance to endure. Yet, treatment? Less — long haul treatment is hard to finish without nonstop help and a long-haul treatment plan. Numerous patients quit going to therapy, bolster gatherings, and take recommended drugs except if they are constrained to follow a set treatment plan and have sufficient backings set up to help keep them on target.

Enslavement is corresponded to an impressive, lessening in an individual's capacity to downgrade or separate from habits learned through the sans model system. This implies problematic substance use influences our ability to settle on choices. As the confusion advances, we start to put less an incentive on long-haul prizes and more incentive on promptly fulfilling a need. Step by step, transient requirements, similar to substance use, abrogate long-haul needs, such as keeping up business or putting resources into individual connections.

For what reason is This Important?

Patients with substance use issues are headed to use regardless of harmful outcomes. Although fixation is seen increasingly more as a procured mind infection, many are as yet bewildered concerning why those enduring can't figure out how to break their "habit." This examination helps encourage a more noteworthy comprehension of the instruments that clarify why. Use might be thought of as "recreational" by the client. Yet, it represents a test to the cerebrum, fortification systems, and prize chains of importance, which can change an individual rapidly and in a manner that is hard for people around them to comprehend. When reward-result affiliations are entrenched—i.e., consuming medications makes an individual "vibe great"— people with substance use issues have changed the most fundamental instruments in their mind and will have more trouble separating from the habitual inclinations.

It isn't clear how individual encounters, hereditary qualities, injury, and different factors change these changes' speed. This examination's aftereffects are predictable with past information portraying how liquor reliance shows a more prominent probability that an individual has habit-based learning techniques over objective coordinated methodologies. Be that as it may, the outcomes do not give us more data about whether natural recuperation is conceivable, and how we could make recuperation almost sure and supportable for patients.

CHAPTER FOUR

HOW KAIZEN CAN HELP WITH CHANGING HABITS

A Good Tool for Long-Term Change

Since Kaizen is more a way of thinking than a particular instrument. Its methodology is found in a wide range of process improvement methods going from Total Quality Management (TQM) to the utilization of representative recommendation boxes. Under kaizen, all representatives are liable for recognizing the holes and wasteful aspects, and everybody, at each level in the association, proposes where improvement can happen. Kaizen focuses on developments in profitability, adequacy, security, and waste decrease, and the individuals who follow the methodology regularly locate a mess more consequently:

- Less waste – stock is utilized all the more productively as are worker abilities.
- People are progressively fulfilled – they directly affect the state of affairs done.
- Improved duty – colleagues have even more a stake in their job and are increasingly disposed to focus on doing a great job.
- Improved maintenance – fulfilled and connected with individuals are bound to remain.
- Improved seriousness – increments in productivity will, in general, add to bring down expenses and more essential items.
- Improved purchaser satisfaction – originating from better items with less blame.
- Improved problem explaining – taking a gander at processes from an arrangements point of view

permits representatives to take care of issues continuously.

- Improved groups – working together to take care of problems helps manufacture and reinforce existing groups.

Another Japanese expression related to kaizen is Muda, which means waste. Kaizen is planned for diminishing waste by taking overproduction, improving quality, being progressively effective, having less idle time, and lessening pointless activities. All these mean cash reserve funds and transform potential misfortunes into benefits.

The kaizen reasoning was created to improve manufacturing processes, and it is one of the components which prompted the achievement of Japanese manufacturing through high caliber and low expenses. In any case, you can pick up the advantages of the kaizen approach in numerous other working situations as well, and at both an individual level or for your entire group or association.

A significant part of the spotlight in kaizen is on lessening "waste," and this waste takes a few structures:

- Movement – moving materials around before further worth can be added to them.
- Time – spent pausing (no worth is being included during this time).
- Defects – which require re-work or must be discarded.
- Over-processing – doing more to the item than is essential to giving the "client" the most extreme cash incentive.
- Variations – delivering bespoke arrangements where a standard one will work similarly also.

The 5S methodology

One approach to approach kaizen is through the 5S

methodology. The 5S's are as per the following:

Sort

Sort alludes to finding and isolating out the things that are a bit much. The objective of arranging is to expel the messiness and guarantee that everything in your condition is useful. While applying kaizen to yourself, this may mean figuring out your work area and evacuating the things that you never again use, similar to old printouts or obsolete manuals.

Arranging organization processes may involve the evacuation of a superfluous advance. For instance, If you have consistently depended on center gatherings when growing new programming, you might have the option to eliminate this progression since you have faithful clients you could study. In the group condition, arranging could occur by getting out shared file organizers, evacuating old gear that is merely laying near, and other comparable improvements. These don't need to be done at the same time, but instead, gradually after some time.

Straighten

Do you or your associates invest a great deal of energy attempting to discover things? Fix alludes to ensuring everything is in a consistent spot, so it tends to be found rapidly and effectively by you and everybody around you. Notwithstanding fixing the physical things around your workspace and aggregate work conditions, advanced fixing should likewise be considered. Are the entirety of your records all together? Will everybody in the group that necessities access to them get to them?

Sparkle

Keeping your physical working condition clean is a piece of the sparkle. It's not just useful for the things around your office or your wellbeing and the general joy of your partners. For instance, the residue can cause hardware disappointment as hypersensitivities. The shape can be unattractive, just as undesirable. Morsels can make consoles stick just as bring pets into your office. Overflowing waste jars can emanate an odor that triggers cerebral pains for delicate individuals. Standard, light measures of cleaning done reliably in a region will guarantee that issues identified with soil and grime are kept away from. Keeping up a calendar of who in your group will be liable for what territories (if a cleaning administration can't be utilized) is the best methodology and will, at last, make everybody neater over the long haul.

Standardize

Standardization, when applied to your processes, can improve things significantly in your efficiency. For instance, you could recommend using a standardized client care stage rather than having the client contact you using support@ email address. That way, everyone can go without much of a stretch track of client assistance issues. Another standardization that can genuinely profit everybody is in the documentation. At whatever point another person gets in your group, it will help them colossally if the methodology they have to follow to do their job is documented. If you can set that up for each colleague in a similar way, it can make onboarding quicker and easier.

Sustain

When everybody in your work condition and your group can proceed with the continual improvement process, they'll receive the rewards. At last, this will guarantee that turmoil doesn't take over in any region of your business, bringing about more joyful workers and more joyful customers. To support kaizen, it's significant that everybody realizes they have a section to play. Everybody understands when to step in If somebody needs assistance or fill in when somebody is no more. Keeping disturbances to continuous improvement insignificant will keep things moving the correct way.

A definitive objective of kaizen is to improve efficiency, quality, confidence, and gainfulness within an organization. When every individual in a group feels an awareness of others' expectations and possession in zones that advantage the group and the organization, everybody will profit. Consider approaches to execute kaizen in your association to perceive what benefits continuous improvements can have in your business.

Utilizing Kaizen as a Tool

Here's our proposed approach for utilizing kaizen thinking all alone or with your group:

1. Keep a thought log of things that appear to be wasteful or that you'd prefer to improve. It's frequently simpler to detect these without giving it much thought than in chilly reflection.
2. Once per month, invest some energy recognizing zones where there is "waste" in how you or your group is working. Utilize your thoughts log as info, yet additionally, consider the more great picture and your general methods for working. Experience every one of the sorts of waste recorded above as a checklist. How could "waste" be eliminated? How could things be improved?
3. Plan out when you're going to roll out these improvements. You have to find some kind of harmony between continuing ahead with making the improvements quickly (so the region of waste doesn't turn into a bigger problem), and keeping

away from "change overload."It is particularly essential to consider the impact or disarray that it could cause other people, which could make them abstain from adopting the change. What's more, a great method to evaluate the impact of changes you are thinking about utilizes the Impact Analysis Tool.

4. If the changes influence others, make sure to counsel them about the new courses of action and tune in to their remarks!

Applying Kaizen to Habit Change

Let's assume you'd prefer to fire getting up an hour sooner. You could move toward this objective in two different ways:

1. Set your caution an hour faster, battle your body's natural inclinations the following morning, and make it slither up in any event when it only needs to rest. After doing this reliably for 30 days, your body, mind, and soul ought to be utilized to it, so it is, in this way, another habit.

2. Or, on the other hand, set your alert two minutes sooner, and when you get up the following morning, you can scarcely feel the distinction. Set it two minutes earlier the next day, in this way, making it four minutes sooner than when you initially began. Odds are, it won't feel too diverse either. Proceed with getting up two minutes sooner every morning, and following 30 days, you're presently awakening an entire hour sooner. Your body was asked to change progressively, and it most likely took its signs somewhat gentler.

Presently, either method could work. I conjecture that it relies upon your character, your phase of life, and how troublesome this potential habit change is. Be that as it may, following three months of attempting the "old school" method of reliably doing a disturbing action with the expectation of it turning into a habit, I think I'll try the "kaizen" way this time.

My objective for habit change

I'm going to perceive how this method works for me. In 30 days, I'd prefer to incorporate practicing three hours per week into my everyday practice. That is 30 minutes per day, with one free day. This implies in one month, and I'd prefer to appreciate the habit of working out three hours that week. The following 30 days is "training" up for that relatively simple objective.

- Week 1, I'd prefer to work out an aggregate of at any rate an hour. That is for 60 minutes. Scarcely anything.
- Week 2, I'd prefer to work out an aggregate of at any rate an hour and a half. One and a half hours. Thoroughly do-capable.
- Week 3, I'd prefer to work out a sum of in any event 120 minutes. Two hours.
- Week 4, I'd prefer to work out a sum of in any event 150 minutes—over two hours.

You'll see the first week is six days with 10 minutes of activity. The subsequent week is 15 minutes – just a short increment. The third week is 20 minutes, six days per week. The most recent week is 25 minutes. Every week is a five-minute day-by-day increment. As I would like to think, a five-minute increase is nothing. However, in 30 days, I'm working out 15 minutes more every day. I'm trusting that in 30 days, I'll have worked as long as 30 minutes every day, six days per week. At that point, I can begin my habit change objective of steady, healthy, gainful exercise.

Your turn

Do you have a habit in your life you'd prefer to supplant?

Does attempting to replace an undesirable habit with a needed one appear to be overpowering some of the time? I realize it does for me. In any case, since habit change ought to be for the long stretch, it merits seeking after methods that produce enduring outcomes. We have to give ourselves effortlessness as we ask after child-rearing, home administration, and being a caring companion, that is, without a doubt — yet we likewise need to respect our Maker with our lives by being acceptable stewards of what He's given us. Think about those seemingly insignificant details in your life that, stacked on one another, form a divider that keeps you from being who you truly need to be.

- Do you need to turn out to be a greater extent, a peruser and a lesser degree a TV watcher? At that point, this month, bit by bit, supplant two hours of TV-watching time with understanding time.
- Do you need to quit drinking pop and drink more water? Continuously supplant your everyday soft drink admission with water until you never again drink soft drink.
- Would you like to hit the sack by 10 p.m. rather than noon? Gradually consider it a night a couple of moments prior every night, until you wind up yawning and prepare to hit the sack by 10.

On Monday, we'll talk increasingly about picking individual goals, yet perhaps you're now in the quest for some self-awareness. In any case — what habit in your life might you want to change? Dream on this throughout the end of the week... And recollect, habit change will, in general, work best when we stay with just one, so seek after the thing most on your mind.

Step by step instructions to Use Kaizen to Improve Your Habits at the Office

Despite whatever your identity is or where you are in life, everybody could utilize a little kaizen, both Chinese and Japanese methods improvement. Kaizen is clarified from numerous points of view, contingent upon the source you pick as your kaizen direct. Right now, going to take a gander at the various ways you can apply kaizen to your expert life and your association.

Where to utilize kaizen

Kaizen is tied in with making continuous improvements within the workplace. These improvements can be made at different levels within your organization. You can begin with kaizen for yourself to make changes that improve your efficiency and joy. Not at all, like other personal growth procedures that expect you to roll out radical improvements, has kaizen urged you to make small ones reliably after some time. Consider it like doing lower than expected trials with yourself.

For instance, you could begin small by going for a brief stroll each day during your lunch break instead of remaining inside. Sooner or later, you can decide to expand that time if you begin seeing advantages on how you feel the remainder of the day. There are many little kaizen-tests you can start your own to improve your expert life. As others observe your changes, they may jump aboard also.

Kaizen can likewise be applied to your organization's processes. Contingent upon the sort of industry you are in, these processes could identify with the manufacturing of an item, improvement of programming, treatment of client care issues, handing-off leads from promoting to deals, getting a corporate endorsement for nearby activities, and other comparative regions. Groups can likewise use kaizen to improve their coordinated effort. In a group, every part is liable for maintaining kaizen principles to guarantee the group's outstanding achievement.

Small Steps to Start Practicing Kaizen Even If You Have A Frenetic Life

Kaizen urges individuals to make infant strides towards bigger goals and focusing on a 1% improvement every day. Similarly, as drops of water can disintegrate stone by diligence, small actions will become significant life changes. Would you say you are prepared to kaizen your life? Here are a few thoughts on the most proficient method to actualize this way of thinking in both your expert and everyday life:

Pose yourself straightforward inquiries

When you have an objective, here and there, you stuck on how might I arrive at it? You see that objective from a far distance and not understanding that it finds a way to make it genuine. Presently, change that mindset. Separate your objective and ask yourself inquiries like "What is the primary thing I can do to make it?" or "Would I be able to put in no time flat daily doing...?" Stick to the idea that nothing comes simple, and it needs a cooperative attitude, tirelessness, and consistency to make your objective materializes.

Make a process

Think of an actionable process for a particular activity that is composed and repeatable. Inspect whether the process is productive by inquiring about whether the process spares you time and If it achieved your ideal outcome. If not, change it. Do not stick in one fixed thing and continue enhancing because our reality is continually evolving.

Organize your actions

Presently you realize the means to accomplish your goals and have the processes set and prepared. Currently, it's an ideal opportunity to choose the request wherein you'll seek after them. In case you're feeling overpowered, start with the action that will be least demanding to execute and go from that point. Back off of yourself, however, stay to do the activities reliably.

Make the vast majority of your time.

If you take a gander at your day-by-day plan, it appears to be challenging to set aside a few moments for yourself to stop and effectively arrive at your objective. Be that as it may, you will require time to make those small strides. Consistently before you rest, review your calendar for the following day and be sensible. Discover a space when you can make some an opportunity to arrive at your fantasy and teach yourself successfully. Do not postpone and state that "best I can do it one more day." If not currently, at that point, when?

Picture

Picture your objective and how you can accomplish it in small advances that you make. Consistently, picture this in your mind, particularly when you start the day toward the beginning of the day. Do not consider the difficulties and hardships; you may look into achieving them. Consider yours to be an enjoyable process that makes you more grounded and better each day.

Monitor your advancement

The idea of kaizen is certifiably not an unexpected, significant change, however small changes that you reliably make day by day. You can record what you do towards your objective every day. Monitoring your advancement will likewise permit you to make modifications varying. Kaizen is a continuous process, so you should continue planning, acting, and altering as you go.

Eliminate waste and overabundance

In your manner, to accomplish your objective, you may discover things that are redundant and tedious. Frequently, stop and assess how much worth every activity adds to your life. If, for instance, heading off to the language courses appears to be excessively tiring and insufficient to you, you might need to consider learning dialects online that are increasingly proficient for you.

These straightforward approaches to practice kaizen should assist you in achieving your goals and develop yourself. It might require some investment to accomplish your ideal outcome, yet it will worth the pause. With kaizen practice, you can do your actual works out while not being so difficult on yourself–production the advancement increasingly attainable and charming.

CHAPTER FIVE

HOW KAIZEN CAN HELP WITH BUILDING HEALTHY HABITS

Kaizen Building Self-Encouragement

You Learned to Crawl Before You Can Walk

What number of babies have you known about that permanently removed their containers from their mouths, put them on a close-by table, jumped out of their dens, and start to walk or run? I don't think about you, yet I haven't known about any. The right arrangement is that the infant figures out how to turn over, start to slither, increases self-assurance enough to stand up, increases somewhat more self-confidence, and makes a stride. Typically the initial step finishes in a minor catastrophe, and the newborn child falls. Yet, the child realizes that, at any rate, it made a beginning.

Generally, the guardians are so thrilled about the endeavor that they are brimming with acclaim and cheer excitedly, even though the infant may not have figured out how to make even a single stride effectively. So the bombed endeavor is overlooked or isn't pondered as a disappointment, yet as a fruitful first endeavor, and the youngster energetically attempts again not long a while later. Regardless of whether the person in question doesn't grow up to run a brief mile, in any event, running is aced.

This represents an intriguing fact regarding why individuals, when all is said in done, and numerous experts and administrators need self-assurance later on in life. A newborn child learning an increasingly adult undertaking, for the most part, has somebody shouting out to him. Yet, regardless of whether he didn't, who's to state that that initial step when he fell was an awful endeavor or a decent one? The problem is, as we get more established, others watch us either with or without perniciousness. Many of these spectators are critical and never neglect to tell us when we do a poor job, less so when we do an adequate one or even a pretty decent one. So we get the possibility that it is never a worthy endeavor.

Be that as it may, it is continuously a worthy endeavor. It took my most youthful child, presently a capable administration expert, very nearly two years to figure out how to talk. I wasn't stressed. It took Einstein right around four years!

Addition Self Confidence through Experience Alone as You "Satisfy Your Obligations"

A few of us, in the end, become fruitful along these lines, and there is nothing amiss with doing this. Then again, actually, it is usually a long and here and their excruciating process. Fundamentally, you enter your work or a calling, do what every other person is doing, work hard, and do your best. Ideally, you stick out, and your endeavors are noted and compensated in the long run. If all works out in the right way and as you progress upward, at each stage, you acquire fearlessness.

In any case, with this method, you get passed up the breezes of destiny. Here and there an advancement, you imagine that you earned goes to another person. Through no shortcoming of your own, you could endure a cutback. Terrible things appear to happen at inconvenient occasions; for example, when you have recently purchased a costly house, are supporting a youngster in school, or when you are more seasoned, and it is increasingly hard to secure another position.

If you endure and are somewhat fortunate, you will likely, in the end, arrive at your goals If they are not very high. However, the process is unsure, requires some investment, and there are no ensures that you will find a workable pace need to go, even in the long run. There is an excellent way.

Assume responsibility for Your Confidence Building

I like this method best. It is quicker and with less hazard than the past way. Also, you have more control. The technique of assuming responsibility that I suggest depends on a fundamental principle. You can create anything about yourself, physical, mental, or otherworldly, by starting with a small test and expanding it after some time. Right now is identified with the moderate "satisfy your obligations" method I talked about already. Then again, it is a lot quicker, less hazardous, and you have ensured results since you are not reliant on another person, just yourself, and you don't lurch and gain from "difficult times." You continue intentionally.

Each artisan since the beginning has practiced kaizen or composed continuous personal growth. What's more, you will be a top maker If you put yourself where your qualities are and If you work on building up your classes. For instance, practice a muscle each day, and consistently it will become bigger and more grounded.

Arnold Schwarzenegger didn't begin with each of those muscles that drove him to win global bodybuilding titles even before turning into an actor or Governor of California.

Nonetheless, by practicing with progressively overwhelming loads each day, his muscles got bigger until, after specific years, he was at best on the planet level. This didn't begin with Arnold. Milo, an old Greek competitor, prepared by lifting a calf consistently and conveying it a short separation. After four years, he was all the while raising the calf. However, the increased undying distinction all through the old world because the "calf" was presently a completely developed bull. I don't think anybody previously or since has pulled off that stunt.

Presently I'm not recommending that you begin lifting a calf consistently to build up your fearlessness, Even though this would do the job. In any case, the principle works for building up your self-assurance in a lot more straightforward and more uncomplicated ways. You should simply settle on the choice that you will make a particular move to build up your fearlessness in a specific zone and afterward to do it. Select a generally simple objective to achieve and continue until you arrive at it. Each time you complete an assignment or goal adequately, celebrate and salute yourself. At that point, set a more significant standard or an increasingly troublesome appointment. It's much the same as training with loads. You develop the measure of weight gradually or run all the more quickly as you build up your quality. After a short time, you'll be doing things that you never figured you could. You will have obtained that fearlessness you have to prevail in whatever you want, and usually, you will succeed!

Congruity among Mind and Body

In our worldwide network, stress and tension are two of the underlying issues that influence individuals on all levels from everyday life to work, connections, and one way individuals actively look to reduce anxiety by building up a genuine mind-body relationship. It is hard to see past our tensions since they are an adapted piece of our condition coming from our powerlessness to live at the time and acknowledge demands that are an integral part of life. It is necessary information that life presents a progression of difficulties. Yet, we are sick outfitted to manage them, and it less usually knew how urgent a mind-body relationship is in forming a consonant life.

As per quantum material science, matter and vitality is very similar at a nuclear level, and since feelings usually are more grounded than physical sensations, the recurrence of your sentiments is the thing that makes a physical partner. With everything taken into account, your body resembles a radar for radio wires and moves vitality to the recurrence of your emotions. Fundamentally, negative considerations can make (physiologically) negative encounters. How you feel inside is regularly anticipated by your contacts, so it is essential to prepare yourself to live a reality through a fresh viewpoint instead of a foolish one. Building up a mind-body agreement is collective energy between the two most central components in your life.

Antiquated hermetic writings have discussed how the mind is a swinging pendulum that can change from condition to condition, state to state, and this twofold affects the body. The average fluctuation of feelings negatively affects our responsiveness state since the projection of inspirational ideas can be intellectually depleting. Second, if our musings instantaneously affect our physical condition, we can control our steady, substantial reactions by restraining the mind and practicing mental force. Mind-body congruity puts the subject in his/her actual nature. There is no utilization to make gains in absolute joy if the immaterial association between the mind and body is left undeveloped.

Shrewd people shape their characters. Stress affects the body and hoses the interaction we have with our actual nature. We need a solid fundamental reason for our psychological wellness, and the mind-body agreement gives us precisely that. Physical exercise and sustenance are demonstrated to reduce mental inebriation through discharging endorphins in the body, making us more joyful. When I do yoga, I am mindfully thinking of utilizing my body as a power of expressive vitality. I usually feel more in control of my mental state, and my nerves unexpectedly appear to be so small and paltry. Studies show that individuals who are presented to nature feel less melancholy and a sleeping disorder accordingly. Condition breeds molding.

One must develop a rich concordance between our psychological and physical states all together lead less problematic lives. Bouncing from liable, disgrace, dread, and uneasiness is intellectually and genuinely debilitating. Regularly our dread of feelings is the thing that makes the feeling itself—for example, the fear of fear. One problem tackling method is the utilization of essential oils, which I have tried to diminish pressure and improve temperaments. The mending estimation of necessary oils is likewise amplified when they are mixed (I use it for a sleeping disorder). Restraining negative contemplations is vital in empowering strengthening. If you need to have control over your body, figure out how to control your mind first. Figuring out how to take full breaths through contracting the stomach is a practical method for keeping up a reasonable musicality. Another way is utilizing a solitary center when practicing and concentrating solely on physical activity, and that's it. This clears the mind and opens up the prefrontal cortex.

In a world that qualities speed and adequacy regardless of anything else, pause for a minute to stop, delay and inquire as to whether you have a mind-body concordance.

Why Harmony between the Body, Mind, and Nature Is So Important To Our Happiness

Seeing the sun in the sky is a ground-breaking image of the interconnectedness of all life. Interestingly, the brain has become an image of how separated we are on an individual level. The body lies between nature and the spirit, supported by the previous and affected by the last mentioned. Life gets excellent and satisfying when the body, mind, and quality are in concordance.

The harmony between the mind and nature has a critical bearing on the strength of the body. How we lead our lives is an expansion of the brain. The brain utilizes the body in a manner that could conceivably be in line with nature. Nature isn't some inaccessible marvels. Like our bodies, we convey a drop of life in any place we go.

If nature is the universe, the body is the microcosm. Quality is life situated, while the mind is individual-arranged, and the mind underestimates growth. When there is a conflict between the brain and nature, we attempt to shape the world after the mind, instead of living in agreement with a higher presence. This is the place the contention starts. Quality eventually wins by recovering the substantial structure.

A massive wave may player the coast. Be that as it may, when the wave collides with the shore, its vitality is lost as water sprinkles onto land, and the wave vanishes for eternity. Interestingly, when extremely delicate waves contact the seashore, they effortlessly subside into the ocean. So also, when the mind compellingly extends itself onto the world like a ruinous wave, it can't recover its original unadulterated self. Be that as it may, if the account is delicate and advances helpful thoughts, keeping up its centeredness within, its vitality is returned. Similarly, as the soft sand endures the worst part of a wave's dangerous power, the body endures under the mind, which harbors negative energies.

Dissimilar to the mind, which does not consistently put forth a concentrated effort to all life, favoring a few and pulverizing others, nature does not work under set inclinations. Change may be seen, by all accounts, to be delayed in the realm of life contrasted with the mind, as they run on various time scales. The soul need not hinder its pace of turnover of considerations. If we dial down our contribution with the mind, we will start to move away from the mind's eager activity. There is profound stillness in nature, as to confirm by the mountains and trees which face the trial of time. Our inward nature is likewise one of silence. Through the mind, we can see the calm in life. However, internal stillness must be experienced through mindfulness.

The mind is sandwiched in the middle of the inward and the external, working like a street divider isolating traffic in inverse ways. The idea of the outside world is unique, and that of the inner world is union. The mind and the faculties are situated towards outward differences, allowing us to appreciate the assortment in nature. Mindfulness carries us to an understanding that vitality's outward dissimilarity and internal intermingling are the equivalents. Getting a charge out of the external world through the mind, while mindfulness is moored in the idea of the unity of everything, brings the mind, body, and nature into perfect equalization.

The mind is given to us as a play area, and from the account, we can go in any case, inwards or outwards. Kids can rapidly abandon the past as they utilize the mind like a play area. Grown-ups transform the mind into battlegrounds where they can't desert the past. All ill will lives in mind. Clashes start in mind for the sake of guarding the past and securing what's to come. The present is overlooked; it is the place the body and nature exist. When we become altogether mind situated, the body and environment become coincidental, and the harmony between the three - mind, body, and soul is lost.

At the point when the parity is lost, the mind is tested through tests. Nature does not clutch anything. However, the brain attempts to grip everything. The preliminaries we face in life are connected to the connection we have to the lesser self or the conscience. The more we are joined to the lower self, the less we can communicate characteristic internal excellence and inventiveness, which all people have. Vitality is ceaselessly flowing within our being. It can show as bliss, ingenuity, love, and empathy: connections slowdown that vitality and cause it to flow around the conscience. Subsequently, it devastates euphoria, inventiveness, love, and sympathy.

The mind is appropriate for the statement of vitality through inventiveness. Inventiveness is the wellspring of what's going on and extraordinary. When inventiveness revolves around the personality, we discover approaches to search out contrasts and see them negatively. Differences need not be an awful thing. The minute we utilize the word 'unique,' we are molded to relate a negative implication. Each is an alternate articulation of a similar vitality. At that point, looking at life will center around the best, gainful utilization of our innovative energy instead of losing it through damaging use.

We work under the supposition that the mind is essential forever. It is substantial for our reality's transactional aspects, yet for encountering genuine joy, the account will either must be set aside or made empty and open. Satisfaction is real and enduring when mindfulness is permitted to make a scaffold between the internal and the external. The mind can fill in as establishing that connection as it is the interface for interaction with the world. Instead of becoming a partitioning factor, the account will transform into a joining consideration when mindfulness blooms. Mindfulness resembles the internal sun. It prepares for us to encounter the interconnectedness of life that the external sun symbolizes.

CHAPTER SIX

HOW KAIZEN CAN HELP IN WORKING LIFE

Organization

Beginning with Kaizen can appear to be overwhelming. There's a nobody-size-fits-all answer for changing organizational culture – each association is one of a kind in its specific manner. Nor is it simple to compose Kaizen Events. Except if there's a great deal of commitment and challenging work from your representatives, the activity won't go far. There are, in any case, a few prescribed procedures that can make the adoption of Kaizen simpler. Since the two aspects of Kaizen are interconnected, we'll spread how to get each going.

Building up a Culture of Kaizen

The initial step to rolling out a genuine improvement to organizational culture is making the declaration. Tell your workers that starting now and into the foreseeable future, you'll be unexpectedly doing things apiece. Clarify that any sort of recommendations for process improvement will be esteemed and compensated. This should, notwithstanding, be reflected in the conduct of your supervisory crew. They ought to never reject offers of help or recommendations for improvement. At that point, you'll have to make sense of an approach to get the process and examine these proposals. As indicated by Masaaki Imai, a Japanese administration specialist, one method to do this is by executing Kaizen Corners.

A Kaizen Corner is where your workers can go to present

their thoughts. In case you're outdated, you can make it an actual spot. Also, you could generally do it online through programming or email. For the execution part, Maasaki prescribes doing it in 3 phases.

- Stage One – All the submitted proposals are considered and assessed. If they're not incorporated, the worker gets input on the "why." This stage guarantees that your representatives realize their supposition is esteemed and won't be debilitated.
- Stage Two – You train the representatives on how process improvement works, permitting them to contribute better.
- Stage Three – Create a prizes system for representatives that genuinely work hard to help with process improvement. Along these lines, the whole activity isn't only a stage that your representatives will get exhausted.

Now and again, however, your usual representative can't assist a lot with process improvement. While they do know their job, they can't help with anything excessively specialized. For any such errand, you would need to utilize a gathering of specialists with a dedicated foundation. When you have the ball moving and have many thoughts on the best way to improve your association, you can begin sorting out Kaizen Events.

Improve Processes with Kaizen Events

Past all the hypotheses and theories, Kaizen is made out of many tools or methodologies that help set up all that as a regular occurrence. The machines are a piece of "Kaizen Events," which implies a process improvement activity in layman's terms. That is the point at which you pinpoint a problem and begin working towards an answer. When you've pinpointed quite a particular issue, you can arrange a Kaizen Event to comprehend it.

The standard strides here are.

- Organize the Team – You'll require a Quality Control Circle (QCC) to help tackle the problem. For the most part, this group comprises a few shop-floor representatives, process pros, and somebody from the administration.
- Pinpoint the Exact Problem – You should be quite specific about this. What's the exact problem you're attempting to illuminate? What's a reasonable result? To make this simpler, you can utilize Business Process Mapping.
- Find Key Metrics – If you don't comprehend what you're improving, the whole activity will waste. Make sense of what measurements to follow and benchmark so you have something to contrast and the new process.
- Create Potential Solutions – This progression, as guaranteed, shifts relying upon what process you're improving. It could mean anything: expelling ventures from a process, adopting new programming, and so forth.
- Test the Solutions – Compare the new measurements to the old. Is the new process performing better? Remember that occasionally, the arrangement can be the present moment. You could, for instance, improve item yield and imperfection rate simultaneously. The first can be seen from the beginning, yet the latter may require a long time to spring up.
- Implement the New Process Company-Wide – Once you're confident that the new process is working superior to the past, you can begin scaling it.

Process Management with Workflow Software

Back in the days of yore, this was done physically. You discover a process to fix, coax it out on a bit of paper, and execute potential improvements. Today, this isn't exactly the most effective choice. There are programming arrangements accessible for pretty much everything. Business process the executives programming (BPMS) is the best partner you can have regarding actualizing Kaizen in your workplace. Such tools help you.

- Changing Processes – Once you've thought of improvements to a process, you have to discuss it with your workers. Except if you just have a bunch of representatives, however, this can be hard. A few representatives may not ultimately see how the new process is done; others may regularly overlook the latest changes. With BPM programming, you should simply change the process within the stage. Therefore, the system will ensure that everybody adheres to the new process.
- Process Enforcement – People detest change. Sometimes, your workers will dismiss or overlook the changes you've made to the process, returning to the old method for doing things. When you change a process with BPMS, however, it's unchangeable.
- Process Analytics and Improvement – Process improvement ought to consistently be founded on information and measurements. You can't improve a process without knowing whether you're doing the job right. Process the executive's programming accompanies inbuilt examination, monitoring any given measurement. Along these lines, it's incredibly simple to track your improvements.

Furthermore, you know what the best part is? From the

process first, board programming is free. Join and perceive how the product can help improve your operations.

Dispensing with Wastage

Waste is all over the place. It influences endless organizations, now and again, without anybody thinking about it. In any case, it doesn't need to change your organization as well. Utilizing Kaizen, you can accomplish a condition of absolute waste disposal and process improvement. Today, we will show you the nuts and bolts of proper waste administration and how to eliminate waste.

The Types of Waste

To see how to eliminate waste for your business, and in this manner, create improvement, it is essential to comprehend the sorts of garbage that influence it. The most widely recognized kinds of waste are:

- Transport – Startup processes and handovers can regularly get drowsy and impeded by waste.
- Inventory – It's critical to deal with your stock, particularly workload. If you don't equitably appropriate work, it can slow down production.
- Movement/Waiting–Simple actions, for example, moving starting with one office then onto the next (even starting with one work area then onto the future!), can add to waste after some time. Sitting tight for partners, providers, and so forth can be similarly wasteful.
- Over-Processing and Overproduction – How much time do you have to spend on each phase of production? Are sure advances superfluous? Over-Processing (improving something that should be expected) can prompt deferral. Likewise, If you convey more than what is requested (or in any event,

going as far as to send something that was not asked!), it could be a waste.

- Defects – Variation, or imperfections, in production can prompt loss of benefit and development of waste, which is why Kaizen, as one with Lean Six Sigma methodology, ought to be utilized to eliminate surrenders they are found and forestall more later on.
- Talent – Talent wasted on work without esteem isn't the ideal approach to improving your organization. Exploit your workers' aptitudes and productively utilized them. Eliminate pointless advances and spotlight on how you can get the best outcomes as a group.

Utilizing Kaizen to Eliminate Waste

You currently know the various kinds of waste, yet how do we eliminate them utilizing Kaizen? Kaizen is a developmental methodology calling for slow, continuous improvement by dispensing with the trash. Keep in mind and it is smarter to improve everything by 1% than only one process with 100%. You can separate Kaizen into the accompanying strides to assist you with bettering see how waste end works:

- Recognize openings – Once you become adept at utilizing Kaizen theory in practice, you will turn out to be progressively mindful of the sorts of waste that influence your organization. Then, you will have the option to perceive, distinguish, and eliminate waste likewise.
- Analyze the process (es) – Scrutinize your production processes. Survey them fundamentally. What is working? What isn't it? How does this influence the remainder of production? What problems would you be able to recognize?
- Develop and test ideal solution(s) – Using the above

information, you would then create inventive answers to help amplify your production. Testing the arrangement may require some investment, expecting you to hinder output for the time being for a more prominent advantage later.

- Study discoveries – Once you have actualized the arrangement, evaluate your findings. Did you improve production, and would you be able to perceive any staying waste yet to be eliminated?
- Standardize solution(s) – Once you're sure that an improvement has been made, you would then be able to standardize your answer. Make sure to ensure you train the workers before executing them over the whole production line. You would then be able to plan for future events to forestall issues.

How Does Kaizen Reduce Waste?

The Kaizen methodology depends on continuous improvement in the office. Utilizing Kaizen implies continually searching for steady enhancements that will assist with improving processes. The final product is intermittently lessening or taking out the waste. These are models that originate from the 8 Wastes of Lean.

- Defects at last item: Improving processes with Kaizen will likewise improve the nature of the item being made. When you can enhance your details, reduce the costs, and convey them quicker, clients will be significantly more fulfilled. Standardized work, a fundamental principle of Kaizen, likewise assists with guaranteeing to manufacture is reliably liberated from surrenders.
- Non-fundamental development: As far as wastes go, movement alludes to any pointless development of hardware, individuals, or apparatus. This may incorporate strolling, lifting, coming to, twisting, extending that all signify time or additional vitality

wasted. When you include cutting-edge workers and utilizing Quality Circles, those who work on the production line each day ought to have the option to recognize zones in their work that would eliminate insignificant development whenever improved.

- Non-used ability: While not recognized by the Toyota Production System, non-used ability, or the waste of human knowledge, has been an expansion to residues' arrangements, changing the 7 Wastes of Lean (TIM WOOD) to the 8 Wastes of Lean. These wastes outcomes from the board not using mastery, experience, and expertise. It can, at last, form into wasteful and stale manufacturing processes. Rather, workplaces that practice Kaizen underline the significance of teamwork and inclusion from all offices.

Generally speaking, dispensing waste will improve by and significant efficiency in the workplace. Kaizen may not create emotional moment results, and it does encourage a situation that energizes and permits continuous improvement. Counting bleeding-edge workers, including chiefs, and recognizing small refinements to reduce waste can be amazingly gainful to an association.

80/20 rule

The 80/20 Principle affirms an inbuilt irregularity among sources of info and yields, causes and outcomes, and exertion and result. It expresses that a minority of cases, data sources, or effort, for the most part, lead to the lion's share of the outcome, yields, or rewards. Business is wasteful. A few assets, be they individuals, factories, or machines, will deliver especially less worth comparative with their expense than will different assets:

- 80% of the surplus is typically produced by 20% of workers;

- 80% of the worth made is probably going to be created in 20% of the time when, through a blend of conditions, the worker works at his/her most significant level of adequacy.

Any enterprise can raise the degree of surplus by lessening the firm's disparity of yield and compensation. You can do it by recognizing the firm's pieces that create the most noteworthy surpluses and fortifying these, giving them more force and assets and, on the other hand, lessening or halting the use of non-performing assets.

80/20 Principle and Quality Improvement

The 80/20 Rule has been one of the 'crucial few' contributions to the quality upheaval, which occurred somewhere in the range of 1950 and 1990. The perception that misfortunes are consistently maldistributed in, for example, how a small level of value characteristics always contributes a high level of the quality misfortune, urged quality practitioners to focus on analyzing a couple of imperfections causing the more significant part of the problems. As indicated by the 80/20 Principle, exertion ought to be centered on managing the 'indispensable few' wellsprings of off-quality items instead of handling all the problems without a moment's delay. If you cure the most essential 20% of your quality holes, you will acknowledge 80% of the advantages.

In Ford Electronic Manufacturing Corporation's quality program that won the Shingo prize, projects have been applied to utilize the 80/20 rule (80% of the worth is spread over 20% of the volume). As much as possible, uses are broken down continually. "Work and overhead execution were supplanted by Manufacturing Cycle Time investigation by-product offering, diminishing item cycle time by 95%."

Applying the 80-20 Rule to Kaizen

I'm partial to the 80-20 principle. Whenever a comprehension of insights, laws of material science, or human science can settle on an everyday dynamic simpler, it's an invite thing. The equivalent is valid in applying the 80-20 rule to kaizen. For what it's worth, and informally, I've seen these things as evident:

20% hypothesis, 80% Gemba - Limit the time spent in the study hall. Evade abuse of PowerPoint. Continue training interactive and hands-on. Make your base of procedure on the shop floor (Gemba) and invest a large portion of your energy there. Discover the wastes, tune in to the individuals who do the job, and roll out physical improvements.

20% reasoning, 80% doing - If you're investing more energy thinking than doing during a kaizen occasion or the "do" period of a kaizen task of longer than seven days. You most likely haven't perused the kaizen venture appropriately or done your homework in the appropriate Toyota Production System tools or kaizen methodologies. The extra time invested in the hypothesis or more energy in the Gemba gathering the facts may help.

20% kaizen week, 80% arrangement and development - If you think the kaizen week itself is the place most of the work is, reconsider. Provision and follow-up are represented as the deciding moment factors for kaizen activity. Legitimate logistics planning, making game plans, characterizing an extension and targets, gathering the information, and ensuring the group is liberated from interferences are generally crucial. Furthermore, Even though you may get 80% of the new condition actualized during the week, staying 20% of the kaizen thoughts should be finished before starting the next venture.

20% of the rest of the action things will take 80% of the fulfillment lead-time. This is a precious thing to recollect when planning assets and finishing dates, making venture courses of events, and so forth to tidy up outstanding action things and bring the new condition after kaizen to an elevated level of culmination. When you perceive this, you'll have the option to stack up on more assets to complete the fundamental way of things and off the beaten path sooner, accelerating the perfect execution.

20% festival, 80% reflection - In request to do kaizen right, you need to commend your triumphs over waste. You have to make it fun. Be careful not to let this escape hand, or begin doing kaizen introductions and festivities for the free pizza. Require significant investment toward the finish of each kaizen to ask, "what worked and why?" and "what would we be able to do better?" If you're not very thrilled about the festival, attempt to persuade others that now things are more regrettable than at any other time.

Additionally, remember that 20% of the colleagues/directors will require 80% of your consideration during kaizen or whenever of significant continuous improvement activity. I could go on; however, it's late where I am.

Kaizen - Weekly Review

If Kaizen's principles feel difficult in law, have confidence that people are designed to look for improvement, which means the more significant part of these principles can be applied instinctively. There are different ways you can begin executing the Kaizen approach in your work-life at present and reviewing them. Regardless of whether you're attempting to be increasingly beneficial at the workplace by lessening interferences or endeavoring to complete an innovative undertaking like composing a book, these tips can assist you with arriving—step by step.

1. Figure out where your time and vitality are wasted.

One of Kaizen's center principles is waste decrease, and it becomes possibly the most critical factor in a more significant number of situations than you may suspect. A vital aspect of opening greater efficiency is to do less, not more.

If you can never discover an opportunity to dedicate to the undertakings imperative to you, it's conceivable that pointless assignments are wasting a portion of your time. Check out what you have to quit doing. We're now and again not mindful of the attentional releases that penetrate our day, so start by reviewing your timetable.

Track each assignment you perform and the time required for half a month. When you have this pool of information, evaluate whether each task is really needed or simply working on autopilot. If you decide an assignment is crucial, how might you do it better or quicker by scaling yourself? Would you be able to make a format for specific reports or messages you compose, for example?

A large number of the pioneers I work with discover this activity as enlightening. They're ready to free themselves from pointless gatherings that don't require their quality or slice out commitments and to-do that aren't creating any substantial outcomes past depleting them.

2. Ask yourself what small advances you can make to be progressively beneficial or productive.

As you begin to distinguish territories for improvement, the key is, to start with, reduced down changes. Think modest. Regularly, our intuition is to pull out all the stops. We get restless and need results, If not medium-term, at that point within a week or a month. However, when you consider that steady improvements after some time are substantially more prone to stick (instead of clearing, destructive changes), beginning small appears to be progressively engaging, Even though it does take tolerance.

If, for instance, you're attempting to support your profitability at the workplace so you don't need to work through lunch, conceptualize what insignificantly problematic changes may assist you with achieving that. Perhaps it implies showing up to work 15 minutes ahead of schedule every morning, so you're not surging, or setting a caution on your telephone to remind you to take a break, making you more reluctant to drive through and disregard your thundering stomach.

If those methods don't have any kind of effect, continue taking a stab at something different. What's more, If they do have any sort of impact, keep on refining your freshly discovered habit gradually.

3. Put aside time to review what's working and what could be improved.

When we get going, we don't set aside an effort to assess what's working and what isn't. Be that as it may, for Kaizen to work, you have to ponder how things are going, particularly when you sense an erosion point.

Like a Toyota representative halting the production line, respite and document focus where your profitability hits a tangle, or you end up getting irritated, baffled, or distracted. Those reactions signal a separate system that should be fixed, yet more critically, a chance to practice discretion and delayed down.

You can actualize an official one-hour weekly review on a Sunday night to organize your concentration and activities for the week ahead. It's critical to find some kind of harmony among enhancement and increase by coordinating both positive and negative encounters. Give a change to the average day by day appreciation practice:

- What was the "high point" of your day?
- What was your "depressed spot" of the day?
- What might you be able to enhance next time?
- What did you feel pleased with today?
- What did you learn?

The outcome of utilizing the Kaizen reasoning

Kaizen is the option in contrast to the sentiments of thrashing and disappointment we experience in the wake of setting excessively aggressive goals or goals, just to abandon them half a month later. And keeping in mind that Kaizen won't change your life medium-term, it can set critical change into a movement—a tiny bit at a time.

CHAPTER SEVEN

HOW KAIZEN CAN HELP IN ACHIEVING GOALS

There is an idea that is typically talked about in business schools called Kaizen. It is generally joined with Total Quality Management (TQM), Six Sigma, Lean Manufacturing, Training Within Industry (TWI), Just-in-Time Manufacturing, Business Process Improvement (BPI), or a large group of other quality improvement systems. While these are fundamentally the same as and share similar roots, Kaizen cannot interpret past the business world into your own life without much of a stretch.

Kaizen adopts a straightforward strategy that centers on continuous improvement. These aren't goliath imaginative advances. They are small, modest improvements that probably won't look significant without anyone else, yet they produce incredible outcomes when joined with a large number of them. Therapists see how compelling Kaizen can be and have composed a few books that jump into the Kaizen practice and why it is powerful. We call attention to the cerebrum's piece answerable for our battle or flight reaction, and for causing dread is the amygdala. Subsequently, one small advance can change your life to make your inquiries short, and you reduce the odds of waking the amygdala and exciting crippling apprehension.

The explanation that Kaizen and numerous other improvement methods depend so intensely on small advances isn't because we are unequipped for significant innovation. It is because we are wired to take a gander at significant changes with distrust and dread. We may choose to begin working out for 3 hours per day; however, our body and our mind are extremely simply enduring it since it won't last. Inevitably we as a whole begin to tire and become unmotivated at the extraordinary exertion we set forth with little outcomes.

By taking a gander at minimal, systematic changes, Kaizen changes our concentration from a significant difference to a small change. That small change, whenever done reliably after some time, will, at that point, become a habit. When it is a habit, it maintains a strategic distance from the battle or flight reaction and gets programmed. This likewise gives us an establishment on which to proceed to improve and develop. We can fuse all the more once we have a solidly settled habit.

Rather than attempting to work out for 3 hours, start by focusing on 3 minutes of activity daily. Locate a predictable time and ensure you do this until it gets programmed and straightforward. When it is more usual to practice for 3 minutes than to skirt the workout, it turns out to be anything but severe to include somewhat more time. By gradually building up to a more drawn-out, great workout time, your body gets acquainted with the activity, and it feels common.

This is so frequently dismissed because the vast majority feel that 3 minutes isn't sufficient. As a general public, we are modified to need results quickly and have appeared after some time that we will face outrageous challenges for right now achievement (for example, weight reduction pills and crash eats less). The brief exercise is the exact inverse of what we will, in general, do. We will, in general, go extraordinary with an unavoidable disappointment approaching. Instead, take a gander at the 3 minutes as a beginning stage. If we take the following three months and spotlight just on the brief exercise, we will probably begin to shape a habit. At that point, we can make the following three months and spotlight on doing 6 minutes of activity. Then, we can go through 3 months and develop it to 10 minutes and afterward 15 minutes. Within a year, we will have another habit of practicing for 15 minutes consistently.

Consolidate that with small strides to improve sustenance. For instance, you are leaving your vehicle far in the parking area to get a couple of more progress, not taking the lift, going to the furthest restroom when at work, and possibly doing ten sit-ups and pushups around evening time. You will probably observe some incredible outcomes. These things, without anyone else, appear to be too small to even think about mattering yet joined; they can be powerful. The matter of fact is that you are building better habits and systems in a manner centered around long-haul achievement, not merely dropping a couple of pounds for summer. I underscored practice right now; it is anything but difficult to identify with for the majority of us who battle with exercise and weight reduction. With no much of a stretch, it can be consolidated into different aspects of our lives, for example, planning our cash, contributing, getting more rest, improving connections, improving as a communicator, stopping smoking, composing a book, and so on.

I would wager that few parts of your lives have just used these principles with extraordinary achievement. If you stop and consider the most significant instruction level, you can see that we experienced a similar process; then again, it was constrained on us right off the bat. We began with exceptionally fundamental instruction and constructed the habit of going to class to learn. We usually started with a half-day and afterward proceeded onward to an entire day of school. We didn't begin with Trigonometry; we started with checking to ten. Every year we manufactured increasingly more on the establishment until we began to arrive at a point where we could, without much of a stretch, peruse and comprehend pages on a book, fundamental math problems, the history of our nation, and so forth. Envision taking somebody with no instruction and attempting to show them the entirety of that right away! It would be overpowering and impractical. However, we expect that when we set goals for ourselves.

Kaizen is a crucial business principle that centers on small strides for development and improvement. In any case, Kaizen can likewise be a powerful method to move toward the things in our own lives that we wish to improve and change. Small advances stay away from the dread reaction and permit us to fabricate a habit that can help us achieve long-haul achievement!

Why You Should Start Using the Kaizen Method to Achieve Your Most Challenging Goals

Other than significantly affecting many lives, every one of these influencers bases their center practices around a compelling yet viable way of thinking that also doubles as a lifestyle. We're talking, obviously, about the Kaizen Method. Kaizen (which signifies "great change" in Japanese) is a lifestyle that accentuates the everyday finish of assignments and gradual achievements that mean a more significant objective.

Nowadays, Kaizen is being utilized as an umbrella term used to portray an entire arrangement of thoughts, popular expressions, and ideas that are intended to improve an organization's way of life and productivity. Also, all things considered: it's a successful way to deal with all degrees of experience. Kaizen is about the consistent improvement of every one of them. It shows you persistence, lowliness, discipline, and the marvels of positive workplace joint effort. Additionally, above all, the mechanics of progress and the significance of association - both in your workplace condition and your psychological space.

If you don't actualize Kaizen's fundamental principles in your own life, you're doing it wrong - customarily. One of Kaizen's establishments is simply the practice of Hansei, signifying "reflection," which is an idea that is established in the focal point of Japanese culture. Hansei is about refining the craft of self-study. It organizes recognizing your very own weaknesses - passionate or something else - and making sense of how to conquer them during the following stage.

Along these lines, Kaizen is centered on improving the individual the same amount as that of the group since they are both very much the same. We've thought of five hints to assist you with adopting the Kaizen path into your life to fabricate a superior you and an excellent "us."

Tricks and Tips

Assemble habits, not mansions in the sky

A meaningful change isn't fabulous, nor is it simple. You can't bounce into a telephone corner and afterward fly pull out as perfect you that you're looking to be, regardless of how advantageous that would be. The actual process of change - advancement, maybe - is repetitive, excess, and exhausting. Most analogies that are utilized to delineate Kaizen spin ideas around working out at the rec center - and all things considered. That is absolutely the sort of mindset you should be in to grasp Kaizen.

Take as much time as is needed - and figure out how to spend it astutely.

Honestly: what's the hurry? If you center on the goal and not the excursion, the outing will feel terrible. If you focus on every one of the means you take, you'll find an entirely different universe of plausibility you're ignoring because you are available. Set aside some effort to layout your objectives as altogether as could be expected in such circumstances. Be as explicit as conceivable about the processes to arrive at these goals will eliminate large waste measures over the long haul.

Fretfulness is reproduced each moment of consistently in our current online culture, and our assumptions regarding how much time significant changes will take have gotten progressively ridiculous accordingly. Requesting prompt outcomes from yourself or those you oversee isn't the appropriate response. That perspective will just make snags and burden things. It will likewise cause the entire dare to appear considerably more incomprehensible.

Instead, decide to figure out how to make the best of the minutes that you have. If you burn through the vast majority of your actual work time, creating an excessive number of spreadsheets or rounding out structures that aren't as pressing or so significant as doing the assignments that will convey quicker you to your definitive objective, ask yourself the meaningful Kaizen inquiry: why? For what reason would you be a deterrent to yourself? On the other hand, If you decide to gobble up time by holding such a large number of gatherings where big thoughts are raised that never entirely appear, assume responsibility for yours. Decide not to make hindrances or waste in your life and the lives of those you are driving. The breaking points your gatherings to one group a day, toward the beginning, and get everybody's contribution about what went right and what required improvement during the earlier day's meeting.

Be that as it may, the lesson of this piece of the story is plan, plan, plan - and afterward plan some more. That way, you're set up for your excursion to a splendid and sparkling future.

"Gradual steps" are better.

Recall how we discussed how all the more fulfilling it is for us to live in the dream of our goals instead of picture actionable plans to get them going? This damages us in different manners than merely distracting us from making sense of minute-to-minute action steps. It compels us into a condition of inaction that has more to do with being overpowered by the sheer size of the work we have removed for us than everything else.

In case you're similar to many people, your past endeavors for improvement have decreased or were drastically dropped because you requested a lot of yourself too soon on (like attempting to fit in three hours at the exercise center on your first day). As a result, you need quick outcomes or feel just as you should do everything simultaneously. This type of mental self-misuse is the thing that Kaizen was intended to resolve.

Rather Than setting yourself up for disappointment by imagining, you can satisfy ridiculous standards that will just worry you and make you defy your plans and make small strides. Do just what you feel good with for whatever length of time that you can remain to do it, when daily, consistently. If you can only welcome yourself to work on your objective for a moment, do that without trashing yourself. Or maybe, highly esteem the fact that you are moving towards what you truly need. Before you know it, you'll be investing increasingly more energy working on your objective as your excitement and self-assurance consistently develop.

Acknowledge your deficiencies and become friends with

them

We, as a whole, have issues. There's no avoiding them. In any case, listen to this: you're the person who finds a good pace they have control over you or not. If you are an ace slowpoke, at that point, distinguish that as a hindrance on your way that you will workaround. Don't concentrate on holding disgrace or blame about it. These feelings will just take care of your inaction. If you approach activities or assignments with a sense of fear or fear since you realize where it counts, they will constrain you to stand up to issues or character defects that you'd preferably imagine aren't there; stop. Be delicate yet taught with yourself. How might you work around them or have them work better for you?

Keep in mind: you can't dispose of what you don't care for about yourself medium-term. You can just acknowledge these things, distinguish them as what they may be, and acclimatized them into your character. Repudiating portions of yourself will just aim disharmony within your mind, making waste and advancing stagnation.

When conceptualizing, be as visual as could reasonably be expected.

Don't hesitate to outline your fantasies, mainly when you're working towards acknowledging them with others. Mind mapping (or idea mapping) may appear to be a shallow activity to a few. However, with regards to driving a group towards a mutual objective, there's nothing increasingly helpful about getting everybody in the same spot. Why? The essential act of truly showing what's gliding around behind the window ornament in the domain of thoughts on a whiteboard, screen, or bit of paper opens up the doorways to plausibility. It gets innovative power that will energize your powerful batteries.

Acknowledge that the excursion never closes

When your work is done, the task is finished, and the objective has been accomplished: what at that point? Do you stop totally, or do you hold changing and descending the street? Will you stay at the pinnacle of the mountain that you've come to, content with what you've done, or will you choose to go on a unique experience and climb the more prominent mountain that allures you not too far off?

If the way to Kaizen is "continuous personal growth," that implies there truly is no last goal on your way to you or your group's definitive advancement. You decide if there is an endpoint. Will you stop your advance and be content with what you've achieved, or will you keep on finding the substantial endowments you can impart to other people?

CONCLUSION

The Kaizen theory expresses that our lifestyle - be it our working life, our public activity, our home life - has the right to be continually improved. Kaizen is tied in with achieving improvements by making small strides rather than exceptional, thorough changes. Even though enhancements under Kaizen are low and steady, the process realizes emotional outcomes after some time. Moreover, Kaizen is a generally safe and economic methodology. It includes process improvements that do not require a considerable capital venture. Thus, Kaizen urges workers to investigate and evaluate new thoughts. If the idea does not work, they can generally return the changes without bringing about enormous expenses.

Past the undeniable advantage of improving processes, Kaizen induces teamwork and proprietorship. Groups assume liability for their work and can make improvements to upgrade their own working experience. Many people need to be fruitful and glad for their work, and Kaizen encourages them to accomplish this while profiting from the association.

When you improve a little every day, big things happen in the long run. When you develop molding a little every day, in the long term, you have a significant improvement in molding. Not tomorrow, not the following day; however, a considerable increase is made in the long run. Don't search for significant, fast improvement. Look for the small growth each day in turn. That is the primary way it occurs — and when it happens, it keeps going.

The Kaizen approach is a reminder that all improvements must be kept up If we wish to make sure about predictable increases. Think about the smallest advance you can take each day that would move you steadily towards your objective. Turning out to be 1% better each day is a straightforward, practical approach to accomplish big goals. 1% appears to be a small sum. Indeed, it is. It's small. It's simple. It's doable.

Furthermore, it's material for most things you need to do or achieve. It feels less scary and is progressively reasonable. It may feel less energizing than pursuing tremendous success. However, its outcomes will be more grounded and increasingly economical.

Kaizen is a long-haul procedure, and the objective is to build up the abilities and certainty of workers. As a procedure, Kaizen works when representatives at all degrees of the organization work together proactively to accomplish ordinary, steady improvements. It consolidates the aggregate abilities within an organization to make a great motor for development. By having the correct system set up, the board can enable its Kaizen to program, gain energy, and succeed. Workers will increase a feeling of responsibility for undertakings and become increasingly engaged with each business aspect. This will, at last, lead to better processes, higher consumer loyalty, and progressively profitable business.

www.ingramcontent.com/pod-product-compliance
Lightning Source LLC
Chambersburg PA
CBHW070110260726
48658CB00001B/65